D0473697

PHYSICAL EXAMINATION & Health Assessment

First Canadian Edition

Carolyn Jarvis, PhD, APN, CNP

Family Nurse Practitioner   and   Adjunct Associate Professor of Nursing
Chestnut Health Systems   School of Nursing
Bloomington, Illinois   Illinois Wesleyan University
                                              Bloomington, Illinois

Canadian Editor

Marian Luctkar-Flude, RN, BScN, MScN

Adjunct Professor
Nursing Laboratory Coordinator
Queen's University School of Nursing
Program Coordinator, Nursing Research Unit
Kingston General Hospital
Kingston, Ontario

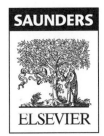

SAUNDERS

ELSEVIER

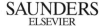

SAUNDERS
ELSEVIER

Library and Archives Canada Cataloguing in Publication

Jarvis, Carolyn
     Student lab manual for physical examination and health assessment / Carolyn Jarvis ; Canadian editor: Marian Luctkar-Flude ; contributors: Annette J. Browne, June MacDonald-Jenkins. — 1st Canadian ed.

Includes index.

ISBN 978-1-897422-24-3

     1. Physical diagnosis. 2. Nursing assessment. 3. Physical diagnosis—Study guides.
4. Nursing assessment—Study guides. I. Browne, Annette J. II. MacDonald-Jenkins, June, 1965–
III. Luctkar-Flude, Marian, 1961– IV. Title. V. Title: Physical examination and health assessment.

RC76.J375 2009   616.07'5   C2008-906108-X

Vice President, Publishing: Ann Millar
Managing Developmental Editor: Tammy Scherer
Managing Production Editor: Roberta A. Spinosa-Millman
Cover, Interior Design: Paula Catalano, Adapted by Olena Sullivan, New Mediatrix
Typesetting and Assembly: Jansom
Printing and Binding: Transcontinental

Elsevier Canada
905 King Street West, 4th Floor
Toronto, ON, Canada M6K 3G9
Phone: 1-866-896-3331
Fax: 1-866-359-9534

Printed in Canada

3 4 5   13 12 11

CONTRIBUTORS

Ian M. Camera, BA, MSN, ND, RN
Associate Professor of Nursing
Holyoke Community College
Holyoke, Massachusetts
*Chapter 28: Reassessment of the
Hospitalized Adult*

Kim Campbell, RM, RN, BScN, MN
Instructor, Midwifery Program
University of British Columbia
Vancouver, British Columbia
Chapter 29: Pregnancy

Dana S. Edge, PhD, RN
Associate Professor, School of Nursing
Queen's University
Kingston, Ontario
*Chapter 2: Developmental Tasks and Health
Promotion Across the Lifespan*

Dianne Groll, PhD, RN, BA, BScH, MScH
Assistant Professor, Department of Psychiatry
Queen's University
Kingston, Ontario
*Chapter 30: Functional Assessment of the
Older Adult*

Joyce K. Keithley, DNSc, RN, FAAN
Professor
Rush University College of Nursing
Chicago, Illinois
Chapter 11: Nutritional Assessment

Shawna Mudd, MSN, CRNP
Certified Registered Nurse Practitioner
Johns Hopkins University School of Medicine
Baltimore, Maryland
Chapter 7: Interpersonal Violence Assessment

Mona Sawhney, RN, MN, ACNP, PhD (Cand.)
Acute Pain Service
Sunnybrook Health Sciences Centre
Toronto, Ontario
Chapter 10: Pain Assessment: The Fifth Vital Sign

Daniel J. Sheridan, PhD, RN, FNE-A, FAAN
Assistant Professor
Johns Hopkins University School of Nursing
Baltimore, Maryland
Chapter 7: Interpersonal Violence Assessment

Julie S. Snyder, MSN, RN, BC
Adjunct Faculty
School of Nursing
Old Dominion University
Norfolk, Virginia
*Chapter 30: Functional Assessment of the
Older Adult*

Rachel E. Spector, PhD, RN, FAAN
Cultural Care Consultant
Needham, Massachusetts
*Chapter 3: Cultural and Social Considerations
in Health Assessment*

Wendy Stanyon, RN, Ed(D)
Assistant Professor, Faculty of Health Sciences
University of Ontario Institute of Technology
Oshawa, Ontario
Chapter 6: Mental Status Assessment

Deborah E. Swenson, MSN, ARNP, CWHCNP
Perinatal Nurse Practitioner
Obstetrix Medical Group of Seattle
Seattle, Washington
Chapter 29: Pregnancy

Denise Tarlier, PhD, MSN, NP(F)
Assistant Professor, School of Nursing
Thompson Rivers University
Kamloops, British Columbia
Chapter 17: Breasts and Regional Lymphatics

Christine Vaillancourt, RD, CDE
Clinical Dietitian
University of Ontario Institute of Technology
Oshawa, Ontario
Chapter 11: Nutritional Assessment

Colleen Varcoe, PhD, RN
Associate Professor and Associate Director,
    Research
School of Nursing, University of British
    Columbia
Vancouver, British Columbia
*Chapter 3: Cultural and Social Considerations in
    Health Assessment;*
and *Chapter 7: Interpersonal Violence Assessment*

Ellen Vogel, PhD, RD, FDC
Assistant Professor, Faculty of Health Sciences
University of Ontario Institute of Technology
Oshawa, Ontario
Chapter 11: Nutritional Assessment

Barbara Wilson-Keates, RN, MS
Sessional Lecturer, School of Nursing
Queen's University
Kingston, Ontario
Chapter 16: Nose, Mouth, and Throat

EDITORIAL ADVISORS

Annette J. Browne, PhD, RN
Associate Professor
New Investigator, Canadian Institutes of
    Health Research
Scholar, Michael Smith Foundation for
    Health Research
School of Nursing
University of British Columbia
Vancouver, British Columbia

June MacDonald-Jenkins, RN, BScN, MSc
Professor, School of Health and Community
    Studies
Durham College
Assistant Adjunct Professor
Faculty of Health Science
University of Ontario Institute of Technology
Oshawa, Ontario

PREFACE

This *Student Laboratory Manual* is intended for you, the student, as a study guide and laboratory manual to accompany the textbook *Physical Examination and Health Assessment,* 1st Canadian edition. You will use it in two places: in your own study area and in the skills laboratory.

As a study guide, this workbook highlights and reinforces the content from the text. Each chapter corresponds to a chapter in the textbook and contains workbook exercises and questions in varying formats that provide the repetition needed to synthesize and master content from the text. Fill out the lab manual chapter and answer the questions before coming to the skills laboratory. This will reinforce your lectures, expose any areas where you have questions for your clinical instructor, and prime you for the skills laboratory/clinical experience.

Once in the skills laboratory, use the *Student Laboratory Manual* as a direct clinical tool. Each chapter contains assessment forms on perforated tear-out pages. Usually you will work in pairs and perform the regional physical examinations on each other under the tutelage of your instructor. As you perform the examination on your peer, you can fill out the write-up sheet and assessment form to be handed in and checked by the instructor.

Features

Each chapter is divided into two parts—cognitive and clinical—and contains:

* Purpose—a brief summary of the material you are learning in this chapter
* Reading Assignment—the corresponding chapter and page numbers from the *Physical Examination and Health Assessment* textbook, and space for your instructor to assign journal articles
* Audio-Visual Assignment—the corresponding video assignment from the Physical Examination and Health Assessment DVD Series, which is adapted from the *Physical Examination and Health Assessment* textbook, as well as space for your instructor to assign relevant audio or computer-assisted learning modules
* Glossary—important and specialized terms from the textbook chapter with accompanying definitions
* Study Guide—specific short-answer and fill-in questions to help you highlight and learn content from the chapter. The critical thinking questions from the video assessment series are included to coordinate the reading and video assignments. Important illustrations of human anatomy have been reproduced from the textbook with the labels deleted so that you can identify and fill in the names of the structures yourself.
* Review Questions—new and revised multiple-choice questions, matching, and short-answer questions in a format similar to usual college classroom examinations, so that you can monitor your own mastery of the material. Take the self-examination when you are ready and then check your answers against the correct answers given in Appendix A.
* Clinical Objectives—behavioural objectives that you should achieve during your peer practice in the regional examinations
* Regional Write-up Sheets—complete yet succinct physical examination forms that you can use in the skills lab or in the clinical setting. These serve as a memory prompt, listing key history questions and physical examination steps, and they serve as a means of recording data during the client encounter.
* Narrative Summary Forms—S O A P format, so that you can learn to chart narrative accounts of the history and physical examination findings. These forms have accompanying sketches of regional anatomy and are an especially useful exercise for those studying for advanced practice roles.

Learning the skills of history taking and physical examination requires two kinds of practice: cognitive and clinical. It is my hope that this *Student Laboratory Manual* will help you achieve both of these learning and practice modalities.

CAROLYN JARVIS

ACKNOWLEDGEMENTS

I am grateful to all those on the team at W.B. Saunders Company (Elsevier) who worked on the *Student Laboratory Manual*. My thanks extend to Robin Carter, Executive Editor, Nursing, for her leadership, encouragement, and organizational support; and to Deanna Davis, Developmental Editor; Mary Parker, Senior Editorial Assistant; and Ann Rogers, Project Manager, for their extreme helpfulness, and for their guidance and coordination in various stages of production.

CAROLYN JARVIS

As Canadian editor, I am grateful for the support of the Elsevier Canada staff, especially the publisher, Ann Millar, and the managing developmental editor, Martina van de Velde. I would also like to thank the Canadian Editorial Advisors, Annette J. Browne and June MacDonald-Jenkins, and all of the Canadian contributors who made the First Canadian Edition of the Jarvis *Physical Examination & Health Assessment* textbook and this *Student Laboratory Manual* possible.

MARIAN LUCTKAR-FLUDE

CONTENTS

Unit 1: Assessment of the Whole Person

1. Critical Thinking in Health Assessment, 1
2. Developmental Tasks and Health Promotion Across the Lifespan, 7
3. Cultural and Social Considerations in Health Assessment, 15
4. The Interview, 19
5. The Complete Health History, 25
6. Mental Status Assessment, 37
7. Interpersonal Violence Assessment, 47

Unit 2: Approach to the Clinical Setting

8. Assessment Techniques and the Clinical Setting, 53
9. General Survey, Measurement, and Vital Signs, 59
10. Pain Assessment: The Fifth Vital Sign, 67
11. Nutritional Assessment, 73

Unit 3: Physical Examination

12. Skin, Hair, and Nails, 83
13. Head, Face, and Neck, Including Regional Lymphatics, 97
14. Eyes, 107
15. Ears, 119
16. Nose, Mouth, and Throat, 129
17. Breasts and Regional Lymphatics, 139
18. Thorax and Lungs, 151
19. Heart and Neck Vessels, 163
20. Peripheral Vascular System and Lymphatic System, 177
21. The Abdomen, 189
22. Musculoskeletal System, 201
23. Neurological System, 215
24. Male Genitourinary System, 229
25. Anus, Rectum, and Prostate, 241
26. Female Genitourinary System, 249

Unit 4: Integration of the Health Assessment

27. The Complete Health Assessment: Putting It All Together, 263
28. Reassessment of the Hospitalized Adult, 273
29. Pregnancy, 281
30. Functional Assessment of the Older Adult, 297

Appendixes

A   Answers to Review Questions, 307
B   Summary of Infant Growth and Development, 313
C   Summary of Toddler Growth, Development, and Health Maintenance, 314
D   Growth, Development, and Health Promotion for Preschoolers, 316
E   Competency Development of the School-Age Child, 318
F   Characteristics of Adolescents, 319
G   Functional Health Patterns Guide, 320

UNIT 1

Assessment of the Whole Person

Chapter One

Critical Thinking in Health Assessment

PURPOSE

This chapter discusses the characteristics of diagnostic reasoning, the nursing process, and critical thinking. This chapter also introduces the concept of health, including the evolving definition of health; helps you to understand that it is the definition of health that determines the kinds of factors that are assessed; and shows you that the amount of data gathered during assessment varies with the person's age, developmental state, physical condition, risk factors, and culture.

READING ASSIGNMENT

Jarvis: *Physical Examination and Health Assessment*, 1st Canadian ed., Chapter 1, pp. 1–12.

GLOSSARY

Study the following terms after reading the corresponding chapter in the text. You should be able to cover the definition on the right and define the term out loud.

Assessment ....the collection of data about an individual's health state

Behavioural model ....moves health beyond treating disease to include secondary and primary preventions with emphasis given to changing behaviours

Biomedical model ....the Western European/North American tradition that views health as the absence of disease

Complete database ....a complete health history and full physical examination

Critical thinking............................simultaneously problem-solving while improving one's own thinking ability

Diagnostic reasoning...................a method of collecting and analyzing clinical information with the following components: (1) attending to initially available cues, (2) formulating diagnostic hypotheses, (3) gathering data relative to the tentative hypotheses, (4) evaluating each hypothesis with the new data collected, and (5) arriving at a final diagnosis

Emergency database.....................rapid collection of the database, often compiled concurrently with life-saving measures

Episodic database.........................one used for a limited or short-term problem; concerns mainly one problem, one cue complex, or one body system

Follow-up database......................used in all settings to monitor progress on short-term or chronic health problems

Health promotion........................a comprehensive social and political process of enabling people to increase control over the determinants of health and therefore improve their health

Medical diagnosis........................used to evaluate the cause and etiology of disease; focus is on the function or malfunction of a specific organ system

Nursing diagnosis........................used to evaluate the response of the whole person to actual or potential health problems

Nursing process...........................a method of collecting and analyzing clinical information with the following components: (1) assessment, (2) diagnosis, (3) outcome identification, (4) planning, (5) implementation, and (6) evaluation

Objective data..............................what the health professional observes by inspecting, palpating, percussing, and auscultating during the physical examination

Relational practice......................recognizes that health, illness, and the meanings they hold for a person are shaped by one's social, cultural, family, historical, and geographical contexts as well as one's age, gender, ability, and so on

Social determinants of health.....the social, economic, and political conditions that shape the health of individuals, families, and communities

Socioenvironmental model.........incorporates sociological and environmental aspects of health as well as biomedical and behavioural ones

Subjective data.............................what the person says about himself or herself during history taking

Wellness..a dynamic process and view of health; a move toward optimal functioning

STUDY GUIDE

After completing the reading assignment, you should be able to answer the following questions in the spaces provided.

1. The steps of the diagnostic reasoning process are listed below. Consider the clinical example given for "cue recognition," and fill in the remaining diagnostic reasoning steps.

Stage	Example
Cue recognition	A.J., 62-year-old male, appears pale, diaphoretic, and anxious
Hypothesis formulation	
Data gathering for hypothesis testing	
Hypothesis evaluation	

2. One of the critical thinking skills is identifying assumptions. Explain how the following statement contains an assumption. How would you get the facts in this situation? *"Ellen, you have to break up with your boyfriend. He is too rough with you. He is no good for you."*

3. Another critical thinking skill involves validation, or checking the accuracy and reliability of data. Describe how you would validate the following data:

Mr. Quinn tells you his weight this morning on the clinic scale was 75 kg.

The primary counsellor tells you Ellen is depressed and angry about being admitted to residential treatment in the clinic.

When auscultating the heart, you hear a blowing, swooshing sound between the first and second heart sounds.

4. Relate each of the following concepts of health to the process of data collection:

biomedical model

behavioural model

socioenvironmental model

health promotion

5. Differentiate **subjective** data from **objective** data by placing an **S** or **O** after each of the following: complaint of sore shoulder ____; unconscious ____; blood in the urine ____; family has just moved to a new area ____; dizziness ____; sore throat ____; earache ____; weight gain ____.

6. How are medical diagnosis and nursing diagnosis similar?

   How are they different?

7. For the following situations, state the type of data collection you would perform (i.e., *complete* database, *episodic* or problem-centred database, *follow-up* database, *emergency* database).
   Barbiturate overdose _____; ambulatory, apparently well individual who presents at outpatient clinic with a rash _____; first visit to a healthcare professional for a "checkup" _____; recently placed on antihypertensive medication _____.

8. Discuss the impact that cultural and socioeconomic diversity of individuals has on the Canadian healthcare system.

9. List three healthcare interactions you have experienced yourself with another person from a culture or ethnicity different from your own. You may have been the patient or the provider—it makes no difference.

10. Using one sentence or group of phrases, how would you describe your own health state to someone you are meeting for the first time?

REVIEW QUESTIONS

This test is for you to check your own mastery of the content. Answers are provided in Appendix A.

1. The concept of health has expanded in the past 40 years. Select the phrase that reflects the most narrow description of health.

    a. the absence of disease
    b. incorporating sociological and environmental aspects of health
    c. changing behaviours and lifestyle
    d. prevention of disease

2. Select the most complete description of a database.

    a. subjective and objective data gathered by a health practitioner from a patient
    b. objective data obtained from a patient through inspection, percussion, palpation, and auscultation
    c. a summary of a patient's record, including laboratory studies
    d. subjective and objective data gathered from a patient plus the results of any diagnostic studies completed

3. Nursing diagnoses, based on assessment of a number of factors, give nurses a common language with which to communicate nursing findings. The best description of a nursing diagnosis is:

    a. an evaluation of the etiology of a disease.
    b. a pattern of coping.
    c. a concise description of actual or potential health problems or of wellness strengths.
    d. the patient's perception of and satisfaction with his or her own health status.

4. Depending on the clinical situation, the nurse may establish one of four kinds of database. An episodic database is described as:

    a. including a complete health history and full physical examination.
    b. concerning mainly one problem.
    c. evaluation of a previously identified problem.
    d. rapid collection of data in conjunction with lifesaving measures.

5. Individuals should be seen at regular intervals for health care. The frequency of these visits:

    a. is most efficient if performed on an annual basis.
    b. is not important. There is no recommendation for the frequency of health care.
    c. varies, depending upon the age of the person.
    d. is based on the practitioner's clinical experience.

6. One of the central skills of relational practice is reflectivity, which is a process of:

    a. enabling people to increase control over the determinants of health and therefore improve their health.
    b. developing a relationship between two persons.
    c. repeating a patient's statement to clarify its meaning.
    d. continually examining how you view and respond to patients based on your own assumptions, cultural and social orientation, past experiences, and so on.

NOTES

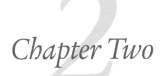

Chapter Two

Developmental Tasks and Health Promotion Across the Lifespan

PURPOSE

This chapter gives a general portrayal of the individual in each stage of the lifespan, considering the physical, psychosocial, cognitive, and behavioural development of the person; presents age-specific clinical preventive healthcare recommendations that detail the screening examination measures, counselling for health promotion, and risk factors for each age-group; and presents a few developmental screening tests used in clinical practice.

READING ASSIGNMENT

Jarvis, *Physical Examination and Health Assessment,* 1st Canadian ed., Chapter 2, pp. 13–34.

GLOSSARY

Study the following terms after reading the corresponding chapter in the text. You should be able to cover the definition on the right and define the term out loud.

Centration...................................the characteristic of focusing on only one aspect of a situation at a time and ignoring other characteristics

Cooperative play ....children playing the same game and interacting while doing it

Delayed imitation ....a child can witness an event, form a mental representation of it, and imitate it later in the absence of the model

Egocentric...................................the characteristic of focusing on one's own interests, needs, and point of view and lacking concern for others

Mental representation...............Piaget's term for the concept acquired by age two years that an infant can think of an external event without actually experiencing it

Object permanence....................Piaget's term for the concept acquired during infancy that objects and people continue to exist even when they are no longer in sight

Prehension................................using the hand and fingers for the act of grasping

Stress..the total of the biologic reactions to an adverse stimulus—whether it be physical, mental, or emotional, internal or external—that tends to disturb the homeostasis of the body

Symbolic function.....................Piaget's term for the concept acquired during childhood in which the child uses symbols to represent people, objects, and events

Telegraphic speech....................speech used by age three or four years in which three- or four-word sentences contain only the essential words

STUDY GUIDE

After completing the reading assignment, you should be able to answer the following questions in the spaces provided.

1. List nine developmental stages, from infancy through late adulthood, and give the general age ranges for each stage.

2. List Erikson's eight stages of ego development that encompass the lifespan, and state the distinct psychological conflict that characterizes each stage.

3. List Piaget's stages of cognitive development in the growing child and state the way of thinking that characterizes each stage.

4. List at least four points of parent counselling that you should include on a periodic health examination for a young child, age two to six years (see Table 2-1, p. 16 in Jarvis, *Physical Examination and Health Assessment,* 1st Canadian ed.).

5. Define toddler lordosis.

6. State four points of physical examination screening you should perform during an infant's periodic health examination, ages birth to 18 months.

7. The preadolescent growth spurt occurs at about age _____ in girls and about age _____ in boys.

8. State at least six points of patient and parent counselling you should include during the periodic health examination for the preadolescent and adolescent years, ages 10 to 19 years.

9. List at least four developmental tasks that characterize the stage of adolescence.

10. List the points of counselling for substance use, sexual practices, and injury prevention that you would include during patient teaching in the periodic health examination of an adolescent, ages 13 to 18 years.

11. List five items of screening certain high-risk groups during a health examination on a *younger* adult, ages 20 to 40 years.

12. List five items of screening for the general population during a health examination on a *middle-aged* adult, ages 40 to 64 years.

13. State the five leading causes of death in older adults, ages 65 years and over.

14. List the screening laboratory and diagnostic procedures that should be performed yearly on older adults, ages 65 years and over.

15. Discuss the implications of conducting a life review, which is one of the developmental tasks confronting older adults.

Note that five tables summarizing growth and development milestones for infancy through adolescence can be found in the appendixes of this Laboratory Manual, for your reference.

REVIEW QUESTIONS

This test is for you to check your own mastery of the content. Answers are provided in Appendix A.

1. Select the best description of the physical growth of an average-term infant during the first year of life.

   a. from 2.3 to 3.2 kg at birth; weight and height double by 1 year
   b. from 2.5 to 4.6 kg at birth; weight and height triple by 1 year
   c. from 2.5 to 4.6 kg at birth; weight triples and height increases 50% by one year
   d. 3.4 kg at birth; weight and height double by one year

2. Human development has been studied by a number of theorists. The best description of Erik Erikson's theory is that it is:

   a. concerned with biological determinants of behaviour.
   b. concerned with the growth of the ego.
   c. concerned with cognitive development in the growing child.
   d. concerned with physiological development from infancy to one year.

3. A game of hide and seek is an example of:

   a. Piaget's object permanence.
   b. Levinson's settling down.
   c. failure to inhibit primitive reflexes.
   d. Erikson's theory of trust versus mistrust.

4. Beth D., age 15 months, has come to the clinic for a well-baby visit. This is the first visit for this child since the family recently relocated. When a developmental history is taken from the mother, she states, "Beth just started to pull herself up to a standing position." The best action on the part of the practitioner is to:

   a. proceed with the examination. The child is progressing at the expected rate.
   b. proceed with the examination. Although the child is behind the anticipated developmental stage, the child is clearly progressing in a cephalocaudal direction.
   c. perform a complete examination, focusing on the musculoskeletal system. Then discuss the findings with the mother.
   d. obtain a more detailed physical development history, then perform the examination. This represents a developmental delay for this child.

5. The use of two-word phrases by a two-year-old is an example of:

   a. biphrase.
   b. holophrase.
   c. telegraphic speech.
   d. ritualism.

6. A group of children are observed interacting while playing the same game. The observer would recognize this as:

   a. parallel play.
   b. language development.
   c. decentration.
   d. cooperative play.

7. The description of alternative periods of structure building and transition in an adult's life are the results of the work of:

   a. Erik Erikson.
   b. National Institutes of Health.
   c. U.S. Preventive Services Task Force.
   d. Daniel Levinson.

8. A life review or a cataloguing of life events is usually associated with the developmental period of:

   a. early adulthood.
   b. middle adulthood.
   c. late adulthood.
   d. grieving for the lost loved one.

9. Tabrina J. is a 17-year-old high school student who arrives for her sports physical. Which of these questions is it most appropriate to ask for counselling in prevention?

   a. How about cigarettes—do you smoke?
   b. How much milk do you drink?
   c. Have you had a flu shot this year?
   d. When was your last vision check?

10. The purpose of the Nipissing District Developmental Screen (NDDS) screening instrument is to:

    a. provide epidemiological data.
    b. form an intelligence test.
    c. detect developmental delays.
    d. reduce risk factors.

11. Disease morbidity is increased in middle adulthood, probably caused most often by:

    a. drinking two alcoholic drinks per day.
    b. obesity.
    c. physical exertion.
    d. stress.

SKILLS LABORATORY/CLINICAL SETTING

You are now ready for the clinical component of mastering the content in this chapter. The purpose of the clinical component is to practise administering the developmental screening tests on a volunteer or a peer and gain some comfort with the tool before administering it on patients of your own.

The Hassles and Uplifts Scale (Table 2-1) is a tool that attempts to quantify the impact of daily life stress on an adult's health. You should take this questionnaire yourself. Be aware that some of the questions are sensitive and considered personal by many people. You should be aware of this when considering whether or not to discuss your own questionnaire with your classmate or faculty member. You will gain considerable insight in taking the test, both on the impact of daily stress on adults and on the amount of daily stress occurring in your own life.

NOTES

Table 2-1   The Hassles and Uplifts Scale

HASSLES are irritants—things that annoy or bother you; they can make you upset or angry. UPLIFTS are events that make you feel good; they can make you joyful, glad, or satisfied. Some hassles and uplifts occur on a fairly regular basis and others are relatively rare. Some have only a slight effect, others have a strong effect.

This questionnaire lists things that can be hassles and uplifts in day-to-day life. You will find that during the course of a day some of these things will have been only a hassle for you and some will have been only an uplift. *Others will have been both a hassle AND an uplift.*

DIRECTIONS: Please think about how much of a hassle and how much of an uplift each item was for you today. Please indicate on the left-hand side of the page (under "HASSLES") how much of a hassle the item was by circling the appropriate number. Then indicate on the right-hand side of the page (under "UPLIFTS") how much of an uplift it was for you by circling the appropriate number.

Remember, circle one number on the left-hand side of the page *and* one number on the right-hand side of the page for *each* item.

PLEASE FILL OUT THIS QUESTIONNAIRE JUST BEFORE YOU GO TO BED.

HASSLES AND UPLIFTS SCALE

How much of a hassle was this item for you today?	How much of an uplift was this item for you today?
HASSLES	UPLIFTS
0 = *None or not applicable*	0 = *None or not applicable*
1 = *Somewhat*	1 = *Somewhat*
2 = *Quite a bit*	2 = *Quite a bit*
3 = *A great deal*	3 = *A great deal*

DIRECTIONS: Please circle one number on the left-hand side and one number on the right-hand side for each item.

0 1 2 3	1. Your child(ren)	0 1 2 3
0 1 2 3	2. Your parents or parents-in-law	0 1 2 3
0 1 2 3	3. Other relative(s)	0 1 2 3
0 1 2 3	4. Your spouse	0 1 2 3
0 1 2 3	5. Time spent with family	0 1 2 3
0 1 2 3	6. Health or well-being of a family member	0 1 2 3
0 1 2 3	7. Sex	0 1 2 3
0 1 2 3	8. Intimacy	0 1 2 3
0 1 2 3	9. Family-related obligations	0 1 2 3
0 1 2 3	10. Your friend(s)	0 1 2 3
0 1 2 3	11. Fellow workers	0 1 2 3
0 1 2 3	12. Clients, customers, patients, etc.	0 1 2 3
0 1 2 3	13. Your supervisor or employer	0 1 2 3

0 1 2 3	14. The nature of your work	0 1 2 3
0 1 2 3	15. Your workload	0 1 2 3
0 1 2 3	16. Your job security	0 1 2 3
0 1 2 3	17. Meeting deadlines or goals on the job	0 1 2 3
0 1 2 3	18. Enough money for necessities (e.g., food, clothing, housing, health care, taxes, insurance)	0 1 2 3
0 1 2 3	19. Enough money for education	0 1 2 3
0 1 2 3	20. Enough money for emergencies	0 1 2 3
0 1 2 3	21. Enough money for extras (e.g., entertainment, recreation, vacations)	0 1 2 3
0 1 2 3	22. Financial care for someone who doesn't live with you	0 1 2 3
0 1 2 3	23. Investments	0 1 2 3
0 1 2 3	24. Your smoking	0 1 2 3
0 1 2 3	25. Your drinking	0 1 2 3
0 1 2 3	26. Mood-altering drugs	0 1 2 3
0 1 2 3	27. Your physical appearance	0 1 2 3
0 1 2 3	28. Contraception	0 1 2 3
0 1 2 3	29. Exercise(s)	0 1 2 3
0 1 2 3	30. Your medical care	0 1 2 3
0 1 2 3	31. Your health	0 1 2 3
0 1 2 3	32. Your physical abilities	0 1 2 3
0 1 2 3	33. The weather	0 1 2 3
0 1 2 3	34. News events	0 1 2 3
0 1 2 3	35. Your environment (e.g., quality of air, noise level, greenery)	0 1 2 3
0 1 2 3	36. Political or social issues	0 1 2 3
0 1 2 3	37. Your neighbourhood (e.g., neighbours, setting)	0 1 2 3
0 1 2 3	38. Conserving (gas, electricity, water, gasoline, etc.)	0 1 2 3
0 1 2 3	39. Pets	0 1 2 3
0 1 2 3	40. Cooking	0 1 2 3
0 1 2 3	41. Housework	0 1 2 3
0 1 2 3	42. Home repairs	0 1 2 3
0 1 2 3	43. Yardwork	0 1 2 3
0 1 2 3	44. Car maintenance	0 1 2 3
0 1 2 3	45. Taking care of paperwork (e.g., paying bills, filling out forms)	0 1 2 3
0 1 2 3	46. Home entertainment (e.g., TV, music, reading)	0 1 2 3
0 1 2 3	47. Amount of free time	0 1 2 3
0 1 2 3	48. Recreation and entertainment outside the home (e.g., movies, sports, eating out, walking)	0 1 2 3
0 1 2 3	49. Eating (at home)	0 1 2 3
0 1 2 3	50. Church or community organizations	0 1 2 3
0 1 2 3	51. Legal matters	0 1 2 3
0 1 2 3	52. Being organized	0 1 2 3
0 1 2 3	53. Social commitments	0 1 2 3

NOTES

3

Cultural and Social Considerations in Health Assessment

PURPOSE

This chapter discusses the ethnocultural and social diversity within the Canadian population. The cultural and social factors that influence health, illness, and access to health care are discussed, and implications requiring consideration in the context of health assessment are identified. Examples of current trends in health, social, and gender inequities are reviewed, and guidelines are provided for assessing culturally based understandings and social and economic contexts shaping people's lives.

READING ASSIGNMENT

Jarvis, *Physical Examination and Health Assessment,* 1st Canadian ed., Chapter 3, pp. 35–50.

GLOSSARY

Study the following terms after reading the corresponding chapter in the text. You should be able to cover the definition on the right and define the term out loud.

Aboriginal peoples...................refers to the indigenous people of Canada, including First Nations, Métis, and Inuit people

Culture ....more than shared beliefs, knowledge, and customs; a constantly shifting process that is lived and created between people within particular social, political, historical, and economic contexts

Culturalism...............................the process of conceptualizing culture in fairly narrow terms, or assuming that people act in particular ways because of their culture

Cultural safety ....the concept whereby healthcare disciplines provide care that takes into account the social, economic, political, and historical factors that shape health and healthcare experiences

Cultural sensitivity ....the idea that healthcare professionals should be sensitive to people's values, beliefs, customs, and practices

Ethnic group ....a group, community, or population that shares some aspects of heritage, geographical location, culture, language, or religion, among other factors

Health inequality ....a generic term used to designate differences, variations, and disparities in the health status of individuals, groups, and populations

Health inequity...........................refers to those inequalities in health that are unnecessary and avoidable, and differences that are considered unfair and unjust

Race...a socially constructed category used to classify humankind according to common ancestry and reliant on differentiation by such physical characteristics such as colour of skin, hair texture, stature, and facial characteristics

Racialization...............................the processes whereby presumed "racial" categories are constructed as different and unequal in ways that lead to social, economic, and political inequities

STUDY GUIDE

After completing the reading assignment, you should be able to answer the following questions in the spaces provided.

1. Describe the main principles of cultural safety.

2. Describe three current trends in the demographic profile of Canada.

3. List five of the standards for culturally, linguistically, and socially appropriate services in health care.

4. Describe the inequities in health status experienced by many Aboriginal people in Canada.

5. Describe the changing trends in patterns of immigration to Canada over the past four decades.

6. Describe three factors that contribute to the pattern of declining health status that is prevalent in non-European immigrants to Canada.

7. List the four major determinants of health and describe their relative impact on health status.

8. List five complementary and alternative health care (CAHC) therapies or healthcare approaches.

9. Describe the four key components of performing a culturally safe health assessment.

REVIEW QUESTIONS

This test is for you to check your own mastery of the content. Answers are provided in Appendix A.

1. Cultural competence involves developing knowledge in all of the following areas, except:

    a. your own personal ethnocultural and social background.
    b. the significance of social, economic, and cultural contexts.
    c. the construction of racial categories.
    d. the culture of the healthcare system.

2. Federal legislation containing the policies and regulations pertaining to First Nations people is:

    a. the *Indian Act*, originally developed in 1976.
    b. the *Indian Act*, originally developed in 1876.
    c. the *Multiculturalism Act*, originally developed in 1985.
    d. the *Aboriginal Act*, originally developed in 1907.

3. The vast majority of recent immigrants to Canada live in the following major cities:

   a. Toronto, Montreal, and Calgary
   b. Toronto, Montreal, and Ottawa
   c. Toronto, Montreal, and Vancouver
   d. Toronto, Vancouver, and Ottawa

4. All of the following statements are true, except:

   a. Poverty is a primary cause of poor health among Canadians.
   b. People who come from the same country will have the same cultural, social, and linguistic backgrounds.
   c. People who immigrate to Canada often experience difficulties getting the help they need from healthcare professionals, hospitals, and other healthcare agencies.
   d. The concept of race has no basis in biological reality.

5. Which of the following groups are more likely to become ill and are less likely to receive appropriate healthcare services:

   a. lone mothers in low-income brackets
   b. older women
   c. people with severe or persistent mental illnesses or addictions
   d. refugees, and some immigrant groups
   e. all of the above

6. All of the following questions convey respect while exploring people's varying health practices, except:

   a. "Which church do you attend?"
   b. "Have you found any treatments or medications that have worked for you in the past?"
   c. "Did you use any special treatments or medicines in your home country that seemed to work for you?"
   d. "Do you have any religious beliefs or practices that you would like me to know about in relation to your health?"

Chapter Four

The Interview

PURPOSE

This chapter discusses the process of communication; presents the techniques of interviewing, including open-ended versus closed questions, the nine types of examiner responses, the ten "traps" of interviewing, and nonverbal skills; and considers variations in technique that are necessary for individuals of different ages, for those with special needs, and for culturally diverse people.

READING ASSIGNMENT

Jarvis, *Physical Examination and Health Assessment,* 1st Canadian ed., Chapter 4, pp. 51–70.

GLOSSARY

Study the following terms after reading the corresponding chapter in the text. You should be able to cover the definition on the right and define the term out loud.

Avoidance language ....the use of euphemisms to avoid reality or to hide feelings

Clarification ....examiner's response used when the patient's word choice is ambiguous or confusing

Closed questions ....questions that ask for specific information, and that elicit a short, one- or two-word answer, a yes or no, or a forced choice

Confrontation ....response in which examiner gives honest feedback about what he or she has seen or felt after observing a certain action, feeling, or statement from a patient

Distancing ....the use of impersonal speech to put space between the self and a threat

Empathy ....viewing the world from the other person's inner frame of reference while remaining yourself; recognizing and accepting the other person's feelings without criticism

Ethnocentrism ....the tendency to view your own way of life as the most desirable, acceptable, or best, and to act in a superior manner to another group or person

Explanation ....examiner's statements that inform the patient; examiner shares factual and objective information

Facilitation...................................examiner's response that encourages the patient to say more, to continue with the story

Geographic privacy....................private room or space with only examiner and patient present

Interpretation ....examiner's statement that is not based on direct observation, but is based on examiner's inference or conclusion; this links events, makes associations, or implies cause

Interview....................................meeting between examiner and patient with the goal of gathering a complete health history

Jargon ....using medical vocabulary with patient in an exclusionary and paternalistic way

Leading question.........................a question that implies that one answer would be better than another

Nonverbal communication.......message conveyed through body language—posture, gestures, facial expression, eye contact, touch, and even where one places the chairs

Open-ended questions...............asks for longer narrative information; unbiased; leaves the person free to answer in any way

Reflection ....examiner response that echoes the patient's words; repeats part of what patient has just said

Summary....................................final review of what examiner understands patient has said; condenses facts and presents a survey of how the examiner perceives the health problem or need

Verbal communication..............messages sent through spoken words, vocalizations, tone of voice

STUDY GUIDE

After completing the reading assignment, you should be able to answer the following questions in the spaces provided.

1. List eight items of information that should be communicated to the patient concerning the terms or expectations of the interview.

2. Describe the points to consider in preparing the physical setting for the interview.

3. List the pros and cons of note-taking during the interview.

4. Contrast open-ended versus closed questions and explain the purpose of each during the interview.

5. List the nine types of examiner responses that could be used during the interview, and give a short example of each.

6. List the ten traps of interviewing, and give a short example of each.

7. State at least seven types of nonverbal behaviours that an interviewer could use.

8. State a useful phrase to use as a closing when ending the interview.

9. Discuss special considerations when interviewing the older adult.

10. Discuss ways you would modify your interviewing technique when working with a hearing-impaired person.

11. Formulate a response you would make to a patient who has spoken to you in ways you interpret as sexually aggressive.

12. Discuss the ways that nonverbal behaviour may vary among people from various ethnocultural or social groups.

13. List at least five points to consider when using an interpreter during an interview.

REVIEW QUESTIONS

This test is for you to check your own mastery of the content. Answers are provided in Appendix A.

1. The practitioner, entering the examining room to meet a patient for the first time, states: "Hello, I'm M.M., and I'm here to gather some information from you and to perform your examination. This will take about 30 minutes. D.D. is a student working with me. If it's all right with you, she will remain during the examination." Which of the following must be added in order to cover all aspects of the interview contract?

   a. a statement regarding confidentiality, patient costs, and the expectation of each person
   b. the purpose of the interview and the role of the examiner
   c. time and place of the interview and a confidentiality statement
   d. an explicit purpose of the interview and a description of the physical examination, including diagnostic studies

2. An accurate understanding of the other person's feelings within a communication context is an example of:

   a. empathy.
   b. liking others.
   c. facilitation.
   d. a nonverbal listening technique.

3. You have come into a patient's room to conduct an admission interview. Because you are expecting a phone call, you stand near the door during the interview. A more appropriate approach would be to:

   a. arrange to have someone page you so you can sit on the side of the bed.
   b. have someone else answer the phone so you can sit facing the patient.
   c. use this approach given the circumstances; it is correct.
   d. arrange for a time free of interruptions until the initial physical examination is complete.

4. Students frequently ask teachers, "May I ask you a question?" This is an example of:

   a. an open-ended question.
   b. a reflective question.
   c. a closed question.
   d. a double-barreled question.

5. During a patient interview, you recognize the need to use interpretation. This verbal response:

   a. is the same as clarification.
   b. is a summary of a statement made by a patient.
   c. is used to focus on a particular aspect of what the patient has just said.
   d. is based on the interviewer's inference from the data that have been presented.

6. A good rule for an interviewer is to:

   a. stop the patient each time something is said that is not understood.
   b. spend more time listening to the patient than talking.
   c. consistently think of your next response so the patient will know you understand him.
   d. use "why" questions to seek clarification of unusual symptoms or behaviour.

7. During an interview, a patient denies having any anxiety. The patient frequently changes position in the chair, holds his arms folded tightly against his chest, and has little eye contact with the interviewer. The interviewer should:

　a. use confrontation to bring the discrepancy between verbal and nonverbal behaviour to the patient's attention.
　b. proceed with the interview. Patients usually are truthful with a healthcare practitioner.
　c. make a mental note to discuss the behaviour after the physical examination is completed.
　d. proceed with the interview and examination as outlined on the agency assessment form. The patient's behaviour is appropriate for the circumstances.

8. Touch should be used during the interview:

　a. only with individuals who speak English.
　b. as a way of establishing contact with the person and communicating empathy.
　c. only with patients of the same sex.
　d. only if the interviewer knows the person well.

9. Children are usually brought for health care by a parent. At about what age should the interviewer begin to question the child him- or herself regarding presenting symptoms?

　a. five
　b. seven
　c. nine
　d. eleven

10. Because of adolescents' developmental level, not all interviewing techniques can be used with them. The two to be avoided are:

　a. facilitation and clarification.
　b. confrontation and explanation.
　c. empathy and interpretations.
　d. silence and reflection.

11. Knowledge of the use of personal space is helpful for the healthcare provider. Personal distance is generally considered to be:

　a. 0 to 0.5 metres.
　b. 0.5 to 1.2 metres.
　c. 1.2 to 3.65 metres.
　d. 3.65 or more metres.

12. Mr. B. tells you, "Everyone here ignores me." You respond, "Ignores you?" This technique is best described as:

　a. clarification.
　b. selective listening.
　c. reflecting.
　d. validation.

13. Active listening skills include all of the following *except:*

　a. taking detailed notes during the interview.
　b. watching for clues in body language.
　c. repeating statements back to the person to make sure you have understood.
　d. asking open-ended questions to explore the person's perspective.
　e. exploring the person's fears about his or her illness.

SKILLS LABORATORY/CLINICAL SETTING

Note that the clinical component of this chapter is the gathering of the complete health history. The history forms are included in Chapter 5.

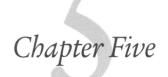

Chapter Five

The Complete Health History

PURPOSE

This chapter helps you to learn the elements of a complete health history, to interview a patient to gather the data for a complete health history, to analyze the patient data, and to record the history accurately.

READING ASSIGNMENT

Jarvis, *Physical Examination and Health Assessment*, 1st Canadian ed., Chapter 5, pp. 71–92.

STUDY GUIDE

After completing the reading assignment, you should be able to answer the following questions in the spaces provided.

1. State the purpose of the complete health history.

2. List and define the critical characteristics used to explore each symptom the patient identifies.

3. Define the elements of the health history: reason for seeking care; present health state or present illness; past personal history and family history; review of systems; functional assessment.

4. Discuss the rationale for obtaining a family history.

5. Discuss the rationale for obtaining a systems review.

6. Describe the items included in a functional assessment.

7. Describe the additions or modifications you would make in environment, pacing, and content when conducting a health history with an older adult.

REVIEW QUESTIONS

This test is for you to check your own mastery of the content. Answers are provided in Appendix A.

1. When reading a medical record, you see the following notation: "Patient states, 'I have had a cold for about a week, and now I am having difficulty breathing.'" This is an example of:

   a. past history.
   b. a review of systems.
   c. a functional assessment.
   d. a reason for seeking care.

2. You have reason to question the reliability of the information being provided by a patient. One way to verify the reliability within the context of the interview is to:

   a. rephrase the same questions later in the interview.
   b. review the patient's previous medical records.
   c. call the person identified as emergency contact to verify data provided.
   d. provide the patient with a printed history to complete and then compare the data provided.

3. The statement "reason for seeking care" has replaced the "chief complaint." This change is significant because:

   a. "chief complaint" is really a diagnostic statement.
   b. the newer term allows another individual to supply the necessary information.
   c. the newer term incorporates wellness needs.
   d. "Reason for seeking care" can incorporate the history of present illness.

4. During an initial interview, the examiner says, "Mrs. J., tell me what you do when your headaches occur." With this question, the examiner is seeking information about:

   a. the patient's perception of the problem.
   b. aggravating or relieving factors.
   c. the frequency of the problem.
   d. the severity of the problem.

5. Which of the following is an appropriate recording of a patient's reason for seeking health care?

   a. angina pectoris, duration 2 hr
   b. substernal pain radiating to left axilla, 1 hr duration
   c. "grabbing" chest pain for 2 hr
   d. pleurisy, 2 days' duration

6. A genogram is useful in showing information concisely. It is used specifically for:

   a. past history.
   b. past health history, specifically hospitalizations.
   c. family history.
   d. the eight characteristics of presenting symptoms.

7. Select the best description of "review of systems" as part of the health history.

   a. the evaluation of the past and present health state of each body system
   b. a documentation of the problem as described by the patient
   c. the recording of the objective findings of the practitioner
   d. a statement that describes the overall health state of the patient

8. Which of the following is considered to be subjective?

   a. temperature of 38.5°C
   b. pulse rate of 96
   c. measured weight loss of 10 kilograms since the previous measurement
   d. pain lasting two hours

9. When taking a health history for a child, what information, in addition to that for an adult, is usually obtained?

   a. coping and stress management
   b. a review of immunizations received
   c. environmental hazards
   d. hospitalization history

10. Functional assessment measures how a person manages day-to-day activities. The impact of a disease on the daily activities of older adults is referred to as:

    a. interpersonal relationship assessment.
    b. instrumental activities of daily living.
    c. reason for seeking care.
    d. disease burden.

SKILLS LABORATORY/CLINICAL SETTING

You are now ready for the clinical component of the interview and health history chapters. The purpose of the clinical component is to practise conducting a complete health history on a peer in the skills laboratory and to achieve the following:

CLINICAL OBJECTIVES

1. Demonstrate knowledge of interviewing skills by arranging a private, quiet, comfortable setting; introduce yourself and state your goals for the interview; pose open-ended and direct questions appropriately; listen to the patient in an attentive, nonjudgemental manner; choose appropriate vocabulary that the patient understands.

2. Demonstrate knowledge of the components of a health history by recording the reason for seeking care in the person's own words; elicit all the critical characteristics to describe the patient's symptom(s); gather pertinent data for the past history, family history, and systems review; identify self-care behaviours and risk factors from the functional assessment.

3. Record the history data accurately and as a reflection of what the patient believes the true health state to be.

INSTRUCTIONS

Work in pairs and obtain a complete health history from a peer. Although you already know each other as student colleagues, play your role straight as "examiner" or "patient" for the best learning experience. Be aware that some of the history questions cover personal content. When you are acting as the patient, you have the right to withhold an answer if you do not feel comfortable with the amount of material you will be asked to divulge. Your own rights to privacy must coexist with the goals of the learning experience.

Familiarize yourself with the following history form and practise phrasing your questions ahead of time. Note that the language on this form is intended as a prompt for the examiner and must be translated into clear and appropriate phrases for the patient. As a beginning examiner, you will need to use one copy of the form as a worksheet during the actual interview and use a fresh copy of the form for your rewritten formal record.

WRITE-UP—HEALTH HISTORY

Date _____

Examiner _____

1. Biographical Data

Name _____ Phone _____

Address _____

Birth date _____ Birthplace _____

Age _____ Gender _____ Marital Status _____ Occupation _____

Ethnocultural background _____ Employer _____

2. Source and Reliability

3. Reason for Seeking Care

4. Present Health or History of Present Illness

5. Past Health

General Health _____

Childhood Illnesses _____

_____

Accidents or Injuries _____

_____

Serious or Chronic Illnesses _____

_____

Hospitalizations _____

_____

Operations _____

_____

Obstetrical History _____

Gravida _____ Term _____ Preterm _____
(# Pregnancies)   (# Term pregnancies)   (# Preterm pregnancies)

Ab/incomplete _____ Children living _____
(# Abortions/Miscarriages)

Course of pregnancy _____
(Date of delivery; length of pregnancy; length of labour; baby's weight and sex; vaginal delivery/Caesarean section; complications; baby's condition)

Immunizations _____

Last examination date _____

Allergies _____ Reaction _____

Current medications _____

_____

6. Family History

Specify:

Heart disease _____   Allergies _____

High blood pressure _____   Asthma _____

Stroke _____   Obesity _____

Diabetes _____   Alcoholism _____

Blood disorders _____   Mental illness _____

Breast cancer _____   Seizure disorder _____

Cancer (other) _____   Kidney disease _____

Sickle cell _____   Tuberculosis _____

Arthritis _____

Construct genogram below.

7. Review of Systems

(Include both past health problems that have been resolved and current problems, including date of onset.)
(Circle if present.)   (Comment, if needed.)

General Overall Health State: Present weight (gain or loss, period of time, by diet or other factors), fatigue, weakness or malaise, fever, chills, sweats, or night sweats.

Skin: History of skin disease (eczema, psoriasis, hives), pigment or colour change, change in mole, excessive dryness or moisture, pruritus, excessive bruising, rash, or lesion.

Hair: Recent loss, change in texture.

Nails: Change in shape, colour, or brittleness.
  Health Promotion: Amount of sun exposure, method of self-care for skin and hair.

Head: Any unusually frequent or severe headache, any head injury, dizziness (syncope), or vertigo.

Eyes: Difficulty with vision (decreased acuity, blurring, blind spots), eye pain, diplopia (double vision), redness or swelling, watering or discharge, glaucoma, or cataracts.
  Health Promotion: Wears glasses or contacts; last vision check or glaucoma test; how coping with loss of vision if any.

Ears: Earaches, infections, discharge and its characteristics, tinnitus, or vertigo.
  Health Promotion: Hearing loss, hearing aid use, how loss affects daily life, any exposure to environmental noise, method of cleaning ears.

Nose and Sinuses: Discharge and its characteristics, any unusually frequent or severe colds, sinus pain, nasal obstruction, nosebleeds, allergies or hay fever, or change in sense of smell.

Mouth and Throat: Mouth pain, frequent sore throat, bleeding gums, toothache, lesion in mouth or tongue, dysphagia, hoarseness or voice change, tonsillectomy, altered taste.
  Health Promotion: Pattern of daily dental care, use of prostheses (dentures, bridge), and last dental checkup.

Neck: Pain, limitation of motion, lumps or swelling, enlarged or tender nodes, goiter.

Breast: Pain, lump, nipple discharge, rash, history of breast disease, any surgery on breasts.
  Axilla: Tenderness, lump or swelling, rash.
  Health Promotion: Performs breast self-examination, including its frequency and method used, last mammogram and results.

Respiratory System: History of lung disease (asthma, emphysema, bronchitis, pneumonia, tuberculosis), chest pain with breathing, wheezing or noisy breathing, shortness of breath, how much activity produces shortness of breath, cough, sputum (colour, amount), hemoptysis, toxin or pollution exposure.

> **Health Promotion:** Last chest X-ray.

Cardiovascular System: Precordial or retrosternal pain, palpitation, cyanosis, dyspnea on exertion (specify amount of exertion it takes to produce dyspnea), orthopnea, paroxysmal nocturnal dyspnea, nocturia, edema, history of heart murmur, hypertension, coronary artery disease, anemia.

> **Health Promotion:** Date of last ECG or other heart tests and results.

Peripheral Vascular System: Coldness, numbness and tingling, swelling of legs (time of day, activity), discoloration in hands or feet (bluish red, pallor, mottling, associated with position, especially around feet and ankles), varicose veins or complications, intermittent claudication, thrombophlebitis, ulcers.

> **Health Promotion:** If work involves long-term sitting or standing, avoid crossing legs at the knees, wear support hose.

Gastrointestinal System: Appetite, food intolerance, dysphagia, heartburn, indigestion, pain (associated with eating), other abdominal pain, pyrosis (esophageal and stomach burning sensation with sour eructation), nausea and vomiting (character), vomiting blood, history of abdominal disease (ulcer, liver or gallbladder, jaundice, appendicitis, colitis), flatulence, frequency of bowel movement, any recent change, stool characteristics, constipation or diarrhea, black stools, rectal bleeding, rectal conditions, hemorrhoids, fistula).

> **Health Promotion:** Use of antacids or laxatives.

Urinary System: Frequency, urgency, nocturia (the number of times the person awakens at night to urinate, recent change), dysuria, polyuria or oliguria, hesitancy or straining, narrowed stream, urine colour (cloudy or presence of hematuria), incontinence, history of urinary disease (kidney disease, kidney stones, urinary tract infections, prostate), pain in flank, groin, suprapubic region, or low back.

> **Health Promotion:** Measures to avoid or treat urinary tract infections, use of Kegel exercises after childbirth.

Male Genital System: Penis or testicular pain, sores or lesions, penile discharge, lumps, hernia.

> **Health Promotion:** Perform testicular self-examination? How frequently?

Female Genital System: Menstrual history (age at menarche, last menstrual period, cycle and duration, any amenorrhea or menorrhagia, premenstrual pain or dysmenorrhea, intermenstrual spotting), vaginal itching, discharge and its characteristics, age at menopause, menopausal signs or symptoms, postmenopausal bleeding.

> **Health Promotion:** Last gynecological checkup, last Pap smear and results.

Sexual Health: Presently in a relationship involving intercourse? Are aspects of sex satisfactory to you and partner, any dyspareunia (for female), any changes in erection or ejaculation (for male), use of contraceptive, is contraceptive method satisfactory? Use of condoms, how frequently? Aware of any contact with partner who has sexually transmitted disease (gonorrhea, herpes, chlamydia, venereal warts, HIV/AIDS, syphilis)?

Musculoskeletal System: History of arthritis or gout. In the joints: pain, stiffness, swelling (location, migratory nature), deformity, limitation of motion, noise with joint motion. In the muscles: any pain, cramps, weakness, gait problems or problems with coordinated activities. In the back: any pain (location and radiation to extremities), stiffness, limitation of motion, or history of back pain or disc disease.

    Health Promotion: How much walking per day. What is the effect of limited range of motion on daily activities, such as on grooming, feeding, toileting, dressing? Any mobility aids used?

Neurological System: History of seizure disorder, stroke, fainting, blackouts. In motor function: weakness, tic or tremor, paralysis, or coordination problems. In sensory function: numbness and tingling (paresthesia). In cognitive function: memory disorder (recent or distant, disorientation). In mental status: any nervousness, mood change, depression, or any history of mental health dysfunction or hallucinations.

Hematological System: Bleeding tendency of skin or mucous membranes, excessive bruising, lymph node swelling, exposure to toxic agents or radiation, blood transfusion and reactions.

Endocrine System: History of diabetes or diabetic symptoms (polyuria, polydipsia, polyphagia), history of thyroid disease, intolerance to heat or cold, change in skin pigmentation or texture, excessive sweating, relationship between appetite and weight, abnormal hair distribution, nervousness, tremors, and need for hormone therapy.

FUNCTIONAL ASSESSMENT (Including Activities of Daily Living)

Self-Esteem, Self-Concept: Education (last grade completed, other significant training) _____

_____

Financial status (income adequate for lifestyle and/or health concerns) _____

_____

Value or belief system (religious practices and perception of personal strengths) _____

_____

Self-care behaviours _____

_____

Activity/Exercise: Daily profile, usual pattern of a typical day _____

_____

Independent or needs assistance with ADLs, feeding, bathing, hygiene, dressing, toileting, bed-to-chair transfer, walking, standing, climbing stairs _____

_____

Leisure activities _____

_____

Exercise pattern (type, amount per day or week, method of warm-up session, method of monitoring body's response to exercise) _____

_____

Other self-care behaviours _____

_____

Sleep/Rest: Sleep patterns, daytime naps, any sleep aids used _____

_____

Other self-care behaviours _____

_____

Nutrition/Elimination: Record 24-hour diet recall _____

_____

_____

Is this menu pattern typical of most days? _____

Who buys food? _____ Who prepares food? _____

Finances adequate for food? _____

Who is present at mealtimes? _____

Other self-care behaviours _____

Interpersonal Relationships/Resources: Describe own role in family _____

_____

How getting along with family, friends, coworkers, classmates _____

_____

Get support with a problem from _____

How much daily time spent alone? _____

Is this pleasurable or isolating? _____

Other self-care behaviours _____

Coping and Stress Management: Describe stresses in life now _____

_____

Change in past year _____

Methods used to relieve stress _____

Are these methods helpful? _____

Personal Habits: Daily intake of caffeine (coffee, tea, colas) _____

_____

Smoke cigarettes? _____   Number of packs per day _____

Daily use for how many years _____   Age started _____

Ever tried to quit? _____   How did it go? _____

Drink alcohol? _____   Date of last alcohol use _____

Amount of alcohol that episode _____

Out of the last 30 days, on how many days was alcohol consumed? _____

Ever had a drinking problem? _____

Any use of street drugs? _____

Marijuana? _____   Cocaine? _____

Crack cocaine? _____   Amphetamines? _____

Barbiturates? _____   LSD? _____

Heroin? _____   Other? _____

Ever been in treatment for drugs or alcohol? _____

Environment/Hazards: Housing and neighbourhood (type of structure, live alone, know neighbours) ___

_____

Safety of area _____

Adequate heat and utilities _____

Access to transportation _____

Involvement in community services _____

Hazards at workplace or home _____

Use of seat belts _____

Travel to or residence in other countries _____

Military service in other countries _____

Self-care behaviours _____

Intimate Partner Violence: How are things at home? Do you feel safe? _____

_____

Ever been emotionally or physically abused by your partner or someone important to you? _____

Ever been hit, slapped, kicked, pushed or shoved, or otherwise physically hurt by your partner or

ex-partner? _____

Partner ever force you into having sex? _____

Are you afraid of your partner or ex-partner? _____

Occupational Health: Please describe your job _____

Work with any health hazards (e.g., asbestos, inhalants, chemicals, repetitive motion)? _____

_____

Any equipment at work designed to reduce your exposure? _____

Any work programs designed to monitor your exposure? _____

Any health problems that you think are related to your job? _____

What do you like or dislike about your job? _____

Perception of Own Health: How do you define health? _____

View of own health now _____

What are your concerns? _____

What do you expect will happen to your health in future? _____

_____

Your health goals _____

Your expectations of nurses, physicians _____

_____

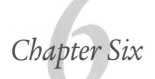

Chapter Six

Mental Status Assessment

PURPOSE

This chapter helps you to learn the components of the mental status examination, including assessing a person's appearance, behaviour, cognitive functions, and thought processes and perceptions, and helps you to understand the rationale and methods of examination of mental status, and to record the assessment accurately.

READING ASSIGNMENT

Jarvis, *Physical Examination and Health Assessment,* 1st Canadian ed., Chapter 6, pp. 93–118.

GLOSSARY

Study the following terms after completing the reading assignment. You should be able to cover the definition on the right and define the term out loud.

Abstract reasoning ....pondering a deeper meaning beyond the concrete and literal

Attention ....concentration, ability to focus on one specific thing

Consciousness ....being aware of one's own existence, feelings, and thoughts and being aware of the environment

Language ....using the voice to communicate one's thoughts and feelings

Memory ....ability to lay down and store experiences and perceptions for later recall

Mood..prolonged display of a person's feelings

Orientation ....awareness of the objective world in relation to the self

Perceptions ....awareness of objects through any of the five senses

Thought content........................*what* the person thinks—specific ideas, beliefs, the use of words

Thought process........................the *way* a person thinks, the logical train of thought

STUDY GUIDE

After completing the reading assignment, you should be able to answer the following questions in the spaces provided.

1. Define the term *mental illness*.

2. List four situations in which it would be necessary to perform a full mental status examination.

3. Explain four factors that could affect a patient's response to the mental status examination but have nothing to do with mental disorders.

4. Distinguish *dysphonia* from *dysarthria*.

5. Define *unilateral neglect*, and state the illness with which it is associated.

6. State convenient ways to assess a person's recent memory within the context of the initial health history.

7. Which mental function is the Four Unrelated Words Test intended to test?

8. List at least three questions you could ask a patient that would screen for suicide ideation.

9. Describe the patient response level of consciousness that would be graded as:

Lethargic or somnolent _____

Obtunded _____

Stupor or semi-coma _____

Coma _____

Delirium _____

10. State the symptoms and physical signs that are characteristic of alcohol withdrawal.

REVIEW QUESTIONS

This test is for you to check your own mastery of the content. Answers are provided in Appendix A.

1. Although a full mental status examination may not be required, the examiner must be aware of the four main headings of the assessment while performing the interview and physical examination. These headings are:

   a. mood, affect, consciousness, and orientation.
   b. memory, attention, thought content, and perceptions.
   c. language, orientation, attention, and abstract reasoning.
   d. appearance, behaviour, cognition, and thought processes.

2. Select the finding that most accurately describes the appearance of a patient.

   a. Tense posture and restless activity. Clothing clean but not appropriate for season; patient wearing T-shirt and shorts in cold weather.
   b. Oriented $\times$ 3. Affect appropriate for circumstances.
   c. Alert and responds to verbal stimuli. Tearful when diagnosis discussed.
   d. Laughing inappropriately, oriented $\times$ 3.

3. The ability to lay down new memories is part of the assessment of cognitive functions. One way to accomplish this is by:

   a. noting whether the patient completes a thought without wandering.
   b. a test of general knowledge.
   c. a description of past medical history.
   d. use of the Four Unrelated Words Test.

4. In order to accurately plan for discharge teaching, additional assessments may be required for the patient with aphasia. This may be accomplished by asking the patient to:

   a. calculate serial sevens.
   b. name his or her grandchildren and their birthdays.
   c. demonstrate word comprehension by naming articles in the room or on the body as you point to them.
   d. interpret a proverb.

5. During an interview with a patient newly diagnosed with a seizure disorder, the patient states, "I plan to be an airline pilot." If the patient continues to have this as a career goal after teaching regarding seizure disorders has been provided, the practitioner might question the patient's:

   a. thought processes.
   b. judgement.
   c. attention span.
   d. recent memory.

6. On a patient's second day in an acute care hospital, the patient complains about the "bugs" on the bed. The bed is clean. This would be an example of altered:

   a. thought process.
   b. orientation.
   c. perception.
   d. higher intellectual function.

7. One way to assess cognitive function and to detect dementia is with:

   a. the Proverb Interpretation Test.
   b. the Mini-Mental State Examination.
   c. the Four Unrelated Words Test.
   d. the Older Adult Behavioural Checklist.

8. The Pediatric Symptom Checklist, completed by a parent, is used to assess the mental status of:

   a. infants.
   b. children ages one to five years.
   c. children ages six to eleven years.
   d. adolescents.

9. A major characteristic of dementia is:

   a. impairment of short- and long-term memory.
   b. hallucinations.
   c. sudden onset of symptoms.
   d. substance-induced.

Match column B with column A.

Column A—Definition	Column B—Type of mood and affect

Column A—Definition

10. _____ Lack of emotional response

11. _____ Loss of identity

12. _____ Excessive well-being

13. _____ Apprehension from the anticipation of a danger whose source is unknown

14. _____ Annoyed, easily provoked

15. _____ Loss of control

16. _____ Sad, gloomy, dejected

17. _____ Rapid shift of emotions

18. _____ Worried about known external danger

Column B—Type of mood and affect

a. Depression

b. Anxiety

c. Flat affect

d. Euphoria

e. Lability

f. Rage

g. Irritability

h. Fear

i. Depersonalization

19. Write a narrative account of a mental status assessment with normal findings.

SKILLS LABORATORY/CLINICAL SETTING

You are now ready for the clinical component of the mental status examination. The purpose of the clinical component is to achieve beginning competency with the administration of the mental status examination and with the supplemental Mini-Mental State Examination.

Practise the steps of the full mental status examination on a peer or a patient in the clinical setting, giving appropriate instructions as you proceed. Formulate ahead of time your questions to pose to the patient. Record your findings using the regional write-up sheet that follows.

Next, practise the steps of the Mini-Mental State Examination, which is a simplified scored form of the cognitive functions found on the full mental status examination. It is used frequently in clinical and research settings.

NOTES

REGIONAL WRITE-UP—MENTAL STATUS EXAMINATION

Date _____

Examiner _____

Patient _____ Age _____ Gender _____

Occupation _____

Mental Status

(Before testing, tell the person the four words you want him or her to remember and to recall in a few minutes, for the Four Unrelated Words Test.)

1. Appearance

   Posture _____
   Body movements _____
   Dress _____
   Grooming and hygiene _____

2. Behaviour

   Level of consciousness _____
   Facial expression _____
   Speech:
      Quality _____
      Pace _____
      Word choice _____
   Mood and affect _____

3. Cognitive Functions

   Orientation:
      Time _____
      Place _____
      Person _____
   Attention span _____
   Recent memory _____
   Remote memory _____
   New learning—Four Unrelated Words Test _____
   Additional testing for aphasia:
      Word comprehension _____
      Reading _____
      Writing _____
   Judgement _____

4. Thought Processes and Perceptions

   Thought processes _____
   Thought content _____
   Perceptions _____
   Suicidal thoughts _____

NOTES

Mini-Mental State Examination (MMSE)

Sample Items

Orientation to Time

"What is the date?"

Registration

"Listen carefully, I am going to say three words. You say them back after I stop. Ready? Here they are . . ."

HOUSE (pause), CAR (pause), LAKE (pause). Now repeat those words back to me." [Repeat up to five times, but score only the first trial.]

Naming

"What is this?" [Point to a pencil or pen.]

Reading

"Please read this and do what it says." [Show examinee the words on the stimulus form.]

(For a full copy of the Mini-Mental State Examination, please see page 101 in Jarvis, *Physical Examination and Health Assessment,* 1st Canadian ed.)

NOTES

Interpersonal Violence Assessment

PURPOSE

This chapter helps you learn about intimate partner violence, elder abuse, and child abuse, including how to assess the extent of the abuse, the extent of physical and psychological harm, including injury, and how to document appropriately.

READING ASSIGNMENT

Jarvis, *Physical Examination and Health Assessment,* 1st Canadian ed., Chapter 7, pp. 119–134.

GLOSSARY

Study the following terms after reading the corresponding chapter in the text. You should be able to cover the definition on the right and define the term out loud.

Child emotional abuse...............any pattern of behaviour that harms a child's emotional development or sense of self-worth. It includes frequent belittling, rejection, threats, and withholding of love and support

Child neglect............................failure to provide for a child's basic needs (physical, educational, medical, and emotional)

Child physical abuse ....physical injury due to punching, beating, kicking, biting, burning, shaking, or otherwise harming a child. Even if the parent or caretaker did not intend to harm the child, such acts are considered abuse when done purposefully

Child sexual abuse.....................includes fondling a child's genitals, incest, penetration, rape, sodomy, indecent exposure, and commercial exploitation through prostitution or the production of pornographic materials

Elder abuse and neglect ....violence, mistreatment, or neglect that older adults living in either private residences or institutions experience at the hands of their spouses, children, other family members, caregivers, service providers, or other individuals in positions of power

**Intimate partner
violence (IPV)**..........................physical or sexual violence (use of physical force) or both, or threat of
such violence; also psychological or emotional abuse or coercive tactics
when there has been prior physical or sexual violence between spouses or
nonmarital partners current or former. ("Partners" includes dating or
boyfriend/girlfriend.)

**Mandatory reporting
of abuse**..a specified group of people (e.g., healthcare providers, social workers) is
required by law to report abuse (of a specified nature against specified
people) to a governmental agency (e.g., protective services, the police)

Psychological abuse ....infliction of emotional or mental anguish by humiliation, coercion, and
threats or lack of social stimulation. Examples include yelling, threats of
harm, threats of withholding basic medical or personal care, and leaving
the person alone for long periods

**Routine, universal screening
for intimate partner violence**....asking all adult patients (usually female patients) whether they have
experienced IPV each time they are in the healthcare system, no matter
what their complaint

STUDY GUIDE

After completing the reading assignment, you should be able to answer the following questions in the
spaces provided.

1. Identify the most common chronic physical health problems that result from intimate partner violence.

2. Identify the most common mental health problems that result from intimate partner violence.

3. Differentiate abuse from neglect.

4. Identify three principles to follow when assessing for intimate partner violence.

5. Identify important elements of assessment for an abused person.

6. List five risk factors associated with homicides in intimate partner violence situations.

7. Discuss bruising in children and how it relates to their developmental level.

8. Identify some of the important elements of the child's medical history when assessing for suspected child maltreatment.

9. Discuss some of the long-term consequences of child maltreatment.

10. Identify risk factors that may contribute to child maltreatment.

ADDITIONAL LEARNING ACTIVITIES

1. Read your daily newspaper for a month, cutting out stories that are related to intimate partner (domestic) violence and elder abuse, including stories about intimate partner or elder homicide, or child maltreatment. Notice the details of the story, including if there is subtle "victim blaming," various myths about abuse that are apparent, or precipitating factors that are identified.

2. Recall whether you were asked about intimate partner violence at your last encounter as a patient in the healthcare system. Check to see if your healthcare professional has any posters about domestic violence or brochures in the restrooms or other accessible areas.

3. Visit your local shelter for domestic violence. Take note of what healthcare services are offered to women and children who are staying there. Take note of volunteer opportunities, and tell your friends about them.

4. Visit your local adult protective services or child protective services office. Find out what happens when a nurse makes a report about elder or child abuse.

REVIEW QUESTIONS

This test is for you to check your own mastery of the content. Answers are provided in Appendix A.

1. Which of the following are examples of intimate partner violence?

   a. an ex-boyfriend stalks his ex-girlfriend
   b. marital rape
   c. hitting a date
   d. all of the above

2. Which one of the following is *not* accurate concerning the challenges associated with routine screening for violence when women come for health care?

   a. There may be potential harm to women from routine screening programs.
   b. Routine screening results in decreased exposure to violence.
   c. Detecting abuse through routine screening does not necessarily result in meaningful responses.
   d. Women may fear that responses from healthcare professionals will increase their risks.

3. Mental health problems associated with intimate partner violence include:

   a. hallucinations.
   b. suicidality.
   c. schizophrenia.
   d. attention deficit/hyperactivity disorder (ADHD).

4. Gynecological problems *not* associated with intimate partner violence include:

   a. pelvic pain.
   b. ovarian cysts.
   c. STDs.
   d. vaginal tearing.

5. Risk factors for intimate partner homicide include:

   a. abuse during pregnancy.
   b. victim substance abuse.
   c. victim unemployment.
   d. history of victim childhood sexual assault.

6. Elder abuse and neglect include:

   a. willful infliction of force.
   b. withholding prescription medications without medical orders.
   c. not replacing broken eyeglasses.
   d. threatening to place someone in a nursing home.
   e. all of the above.

7. When assessing an injury on a child, which of the following should be considered?

   a. the child's developmental level
   b. the child's medical and medication history
   c. the history of how the injury occurred
   d. all of the above

8. Known risk factors for child maltreatment include which of the following?

   a. substance abuse
   b. intimate partner violence
   c. physical disability or mental retardation in the child
   d. all of the above

9. Bruising in a noncruising child:

   a. is a common finding from normal infant activity.
   b. needs to be further evaluated for either an abusive or medical explanation.
   c. is commonly seen on the buttocks.
   d. cannot be reported until after a full medical evaluation.

NOTES

UNIT 2

Approach to the Clinical Setting

Chapter Eight

Assessment Techniques and the Clinical Setting

This chapter helps you to learn the assessment techniques of inspection, palpation, percussion, and auscultation; to learn the items of equipment needed for a complete physical examination; and to consider age-specific modifications you would make for the examination of individuals throughout the life cycle.

READING ASSIGNMENT

Jarvis, *Physical Examination and Health Assessment*, 1st Canadian ed., Chapter 8, pp. 135–148.

GLOSSARY

Study the following terms after completing the reading assignment. You should be able to cover the definition on the right and define the term out loud.

Amplitude ....(or intensity) how loud or soft a sound is

Duration....................................the length of time a note lingers

Nosocomial infection ....an infection acquired during hospitalization

Ophthalmoscope........................an instrument that illuminates the internal eye structures, enabling the examiner to look through the pupil at the fundus (background) of the eye

Otoscope.......................................an instrument that illuminates the ear canal, enabling the examiner to look at the ear canal and tympanic membrane

Pitch...(or frequency) the number of vibrations (or cycles) per second of a note

Quality.......................................(or timbre) a subjective difference in a sound due to the sound's distinctive overtones

STUDY GUIDE

After completing the reading assignment, you should be able to answer the following questions in the spaces provided.

1. Define and describe the technique of the four physical examination skills:

   Inspection _____

   Palpation _____

   Percussion _____

   Auscultation _____

2. Define the characteristics of the following percussion notes:

	Pitch	Amplitude	Quality	Duration
Resonant				
Hyperresonant				
Tympany				
Dull				
Flat				

3. Differentiate direct percussion from indirect percussion.

4. Relate the parts of the hands to palpation techniques used in assessment.

5. Differentiate between light, deep, and bimanual palpation.

6. List the two endpieces of the stethoscope and the conditions for which each is best suited.

7. Describe the environmental conditions to consider in preparing the examination setting.

8. List 20 basic items of equipment necessary to conduct a complete screening physical examination on an adult.

9. Describe your own preparation as you encounter the patient for examination: your own dress, your demeanour, safety and universal precautions, sequence of examination steps, and instructions to patient.

10. What age-specific considerations would you make for the examination of the:

Infant? _____

Toddler? _____

Preschooler? _____

School-age child? _____

Adolescent? _____

Older adult? _____

Acutely ill person? _____

REVIEW QUESTIONS

This test is for you to check your own mastery of the content. Answers are provided in Appendix A.

1. Various parts of the hands are used during palpation. The part of the hand used for the assessment of vibration is (are) the:

   a. fingertips.
   b. index finger and thumb in opposition.
   c. dorsa of the hand.
   d. ulnar surface of the hand.

2. When performing indirect percussion, the stationary finger is struck:

   a. at the ulnar surface.
   b. at the middle joint.
   c. at the distal interphalangeal joint.
   d. wherever it is in contact with the skin.

3. The best description of the pitch of a sound wave obtained by percussion is:

   a. the intensity of the sound.
   b. the number of vibrations per second.
   c. the length of time the note lingers.
   d. the overtones of the note.

4. The bell of the stethoscope:

   a. is used for soft, low-pitched sounds.
   b. is used for high-pitched sounds.
   c. is held firmly against the skin.
   d. magnifies sound.

5. The ophthalmoscope has five apertures. Which aperture would be used to assess the eyes of a patient with undilated pupils?

   a. grid
   b. slit
   c. small
   d. large

6. At the conclusion of the examination, the examiner should:

   a. document findings before leaving the examining room.
   b. have findings confirmed by another practitioner.
   c. relate objective findings to the subjective findings for accuracy.
   d. summarize findings to the patient.

7. When the practitioner enters the examining room the infant patient is asleep. The practitioner would best start the examination with:

   a. height and weight.
   b. blood pressure.
   c. heart, lung, and abdomen.
   d. temperature.

8. The sequence of an examination changes from beginning with the thorax to that of head to toe with what age child?

   a. the infant
   b. the preschool child
   c. the school-aged child
   d. the adolescent

SKILLS LABORATORY/CLINICAL SETTING

Note that the clinical component of this chapter is combined with Chapter 9. Instructions and regional write-up forms are listed at the end of Chapter 9.

NOTES

NOTES

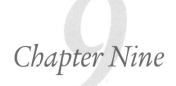

Chapter Nine

General Survey, Measurement, and Vital Signs

PURPOSE

This chapter helps you to learn the method of gathering data for a general survey on a patient and the techniques for measuring height, weight, and vital signs.

READING ASSIGNMENT

Jarvis, *Physical Examination and Health Assessment,* 1st Canadian ed., Chapter 9, pp. 149–180.

GLOSSARY

Study the following terms after completing the reading assignment. You should be able to cover the definition on the right and define the term out loud.

Auscultatory gap .... a brief time period when Korotkoff's sounds disappear during auscultation of blood pressure; common with hypertension

Bradycardia .... heart rate <60 beats per minute in the adult

Sphygmomanometer .... instrument for measuring arterial blood pressure

Stroke volume .... amount of blood pumped out of the heart with each heartbeat

Tachycardia .... heart rate of >100 beats per minute in the adult

STUDY GUIDE

After completing the reading assignment, you should be able to answer the following questions in the spaces provided.

1. List the significant information considered in each of the four areas of a general survey—physical appearance, body structure, mobility, and behaviour.

2. Describe the normal posture and body build.

    height within normal range for posture
    weight within normal range for height and body build (BMI)
    standing comfortably erect is appropriate for age

3. Note aspects of normal gait.

    base width equal to shoulder width
    accurate foot placement
    smooth even and well balanced walk

4. Describe the clinical appearance of the following variations in stature:

    Hypopituitary dwarfism _____

    Gigantism _____

    Acromegaly _____

    Achondroplastic dwarfism _____

    Marfan's syndrome _____

    Endogenous obesity (Cushing's syndrome) _____

    Anorexia nervosa _____

5. State the normal weight range for an adult who is 175 cm tall. _____

6. For serial weight measurements, what time of day would you instruct the person to have the weight measured? _____

7. Describe the technique for measuring head circumference and chest circumference on an infant.

8. What changes in height and in weight distribution would you expect for an adult in his or her 70s and 80s?

9. Describe the tympanic membrane thermometer, and compare its use to other forms of temperature measurement.

10. Describe four qualities to consider when assessing the pulse.

Rate
Rhythm
Force
equality

11. Relate the qualities of normal respirations to the appropriate approach to counting them.

Normally Patients breathing is related, regular, automatic and silent
- most people are unaware of their breathing

12. Define and describe the relationships among the terms *blood pressure, systolic pressure, diastolic pressure, pulse pressure,* and *mean arterial pressure.*

- Blood pressure, force of blood pushing against the well of vessel
- Systolic pressure is ventricular contraction and maximum pressure felt

13. List factors that affect blood pressure.

14. Relate the use of an improperly sized blood pressure cuff to the possible findings that may be obtained.

15. Explain the significance of phase I, phase IV, and phase V Korotkoff's sounds during blood pressure measurement.

16. State the expected range for oral temperature, pulse, respirations, and blood pressure for an apparently healthy 20-year-old adult.

35.8 - 37.3 °C

60 - 100 bpm

12 - 20 bpm

120/80

17. List the parameters of prehypertension, stage 1 hypertension, and stage 2 hypertension.

REVIEW QUESTIONS

This test is for you to check your own mastery of the content. Answers are provided in Appendix A.

1. The four areas to consider during the general survey are:
   a. ethnicity, sex, age, and socioeconomic status.
   b. physical appearance, sex, ethnicity, and affect.
   c. dress, affect, nonverbal behaviour, and mobility.
   d. physical appearance, body structure, mobility, and behaviour.

2. During the general survey part of the examination, gait is assessed. When walking, the base is usually:
   a. varied, depending upon the height of the person.
   b. equal to the length of the arm.
   c. as wide as the shoulder width.
   d. half of the height of the person.

3. A child, 18 months of age, is brought in for a health screening visit. To assess the height of the child:

   a. use a tape measure.
   b. use a horizontal measuring board.
   c. have the child stand on the upright scale.
   d. measure arm span to estimate height.

4. B.D. was delivered by Caesarean section at 38 weeks of gestation because of fetal distress. She weighed 2.8 kg. This weight:

   a. is appropriate for gestational age.
   b. is small for gestational age.
   c. is large for gestational age.
   d. cannot be determined from available data.

5. During the eighth and ninth decades of life, what changes occur in height and weight?

   a. both increase
   b. weight increases, height decreases
   c. both decrease
   d. both remain the same as during the 70s

6. During an initial home visit, the patient's temperature is noted to be 36.3°C. This temperature:

   a. cannot be evaluated without a knowledge of the person's age.
   b. is below normal. The person should be assessed for possible hypothermia.
   c. should be retaken by the rectal route, since this best reflects core body temperature.
   d. should be re-evaluated at the next visit before a decision is made.

7. Select the best description of an accurate assessment of a patient's pulse.

   a. Count for 15 seconds if pulse is regular.
   b. Begin counting with 0; count for 30 seconds.
   c. Count for 30 seconds and multiply by 2 for all cases.
   d. Count for 1 full minute; begin counting with 0.

8. After assessing the patient's pulse, the practitioner determines it to be "normal." This would be recorded as:

   a. 3+.
   b. 2+.
   c. 1+.
   d. 0.

9. Select the best description of an accurate assessment of a patient's respirations.

   a. Count for a full minute before taking the pulse.
   b. Count for 15 seconds and multiply by four.
   c. Count after informing the patient where you are in the assessment process.
   d. Count for 30 seconds following pulse assessment.

10. Pulse pressure is:

   a. the difference between the systolic and diastolic pressure.
   b. a reflection of the viscosity of the blood.
   c. another way to express the systolic pressure.
   d. a measure of vasoconstriction.

11. The examiner is going to assess for coarctation of the aorta. In an individual with coarctation the thigh pressure would be:

   a. higher than in the arm.
   b. equal to that in the arm.
   c. There is no constant relationship. Findings are highly individual.
   d. lower than in the arm.

12. Mean arterial pressure is:

   a. the arithmetic average of systolic and diastolic pressures.
   b. the driving force of blood during systole.
   c. diastolic pressure plus one third pulse pressure.
   d. corresponding to phase III Korotkoff's.

SKILLS LABORATORY/CLINICAL SETTING

You are now ready for the clinical component of Chapters 8 and 9. The purpose of the clinical component is to observe and describe the regional examination on a peer in the skills laboratory and to achieve the following:

CLINICAL OBJECTIVES

1. Observe and describe the significant characteristics of a general survey.

2. Measure height and weight and determine if findings are within normal range.

3. Gather vital signs data.

4. Record the physical examination findings accurately.

INSTRUCTIONS

Set up your section of the skills laboratory for a complete physical examination, attending to proper lighting, tables, and linen. Gather all equipment you will need for a complete physical examination, and make sure you are familiar with its mechanical operation. You will not use all the equipment today, but you will use it during the course of the semester, and this is the time to have it checked out.

Practise the steps of gathering data for a general survey, for height and weight, and vital signs on a peer. Record your findings using the regional write-up sheet that follows. The first section of the sheet is intended as a worksheet. It includes points for you to note that add up to the general survey. The bottom of the sheet has instructions for you to write the general survey statement; this is the topic sentence that will serve as an introduction for the complete physical examination write-up (see Jarvis, 1st Canadian ed., p. 175 for an example).

NOTES

REGIONAL WRITE-UP—GENERAL SURVEY, VITAL SIGNS

Date _____

Examiner _____

Patient _____ Age _____ Gender _____

Occupation _____

I. Physical Examination
A. General survey
1. Physical appearance

   Age _____

   Gender _____

   Level of consciousness _____

   Skin colour _____

   Facial features _____

2. Body structure

   Stature _____

   Nutrition _____

   Symmetry _____

   Posture _____

   Position _____

   Body build, contour _____

   Any physical deformity _____

3. Mobility

   Gait _____

   Range of motion _____

4. Behaviour

   Facial expression _____

   Mood and affect _____

   Speech _____

   Dress _____

   Personal hygiene _____

B. Measurement

1. Height _____ cm

2. Weight _____ kg

3. Body mass index _____

4. Waist circumference _____ cm

5. Waist ratio _____

C. Vital signs

1. Temperature _____

2. Pulse

   Rate _____

   Rhythm _____

3. Respirations _____

4. Blood pressure: R arm _____ L arm _____

Summary

(Write a summary of the general survey, including height, weight, and vital signs. This will serve as an introduction for the complete physical examination write-up.)

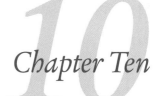

Chapter Ten

Pain Assessment: The Fifth Vital Sign

PURPOSE

This chapter helps you to learn the structure and function of pain pathways, to understand the process of nociception, to understand the rationale and methods of pain assessment, and to accurately record the findings.

READING ASSIGNMENT

Jarvis, *Physical Examination and Health Assessment,* 1st Canadian ed., Chapter 10, pp. 181–194.

GLOSSARY

Study the following terms after completing the reading assignment. You should be able to cover the definition on the right and define the term out loud.

Cutaneous pain...........................pain originating from skin surface or subcutaneous structures

Modulation ....pain message is inhibited during this last phase of nociception

Neuropathic pain ....abnormal processing of pain message; burning, shooting in nature

Nociception...............................process whereby noxious stimuli are perceived as pain

Nociceptors ....specialized nerve endings that detect painful sensations

Pain.."An unpleasant sensory and emotional experience associated with actual or potential tissue damage, or described in terms of such damage. Pain is always subjective." (American Pain Society)

Perception.................................conscious awareness of a painful sensation

Referred pain ....pain felt at a particular site, but that originates from another location

Somatic pain ....originating from muscle, bone, joints, tendons, or blood vessels

Transduction ....first phase of nociception whereby the painful stimulus is changed into an action potential

Transmission ....second phase of nociception whereby the pain impulse moves from the spinal cord to the brain

Visceral pain ....originating from interior organs such as the gallbladder or stomach

STUDY GUIDE

After completing the reading assignment, you should be able to answer the following questions in the spaces provided.

1. Describe the process of nociception using the four phases of:

    Transduction

    Transmission

    Perception

    Modulation

2. Identify the differences between nociceptive and neuropathic pain.

3. List various sources of pain.

4. Explain how acute and persistent pain differ in terms of nonverbal behaviours.

5. Identify the most reliable indicator of a person's pain.

The patients self report

6. Recall eight questions for an initial pain assessment. (PQRStu)
Does your pain increase with movement or activity?
what provokes it?
where does it hurt?
what does it feel like?
how bad does it hurt? (0-10)
when does it hurt
how did it happen

7. Select pain assessment tools that are appropriate for adults, children, infants, and premature infants.

8. Describe physical examination findings that may indicate pain.

Skin and tissue colour, swelling, masses, or deformity

9. Recall how poorly controlled acute and chronic pain adversely affects physiological, social, and cognitive functioning.

CRITICAL THINKING QUESTIONS

1. What conditions are more likely to produce pain in the older adult?

2. How would you modify your examination when the patient reports having abdominal pain?

3. How would you assess for pain in an individual with dementia?

4. What would you say to someone who tells you that infants do not remember pain and that they are too little for the pain to have any damaging effect?

5. What would you say to a colleague who remarks that the individual with Alzheimer's disease does not feel pain and therefore does not require an analgesic?

Fill in the labels indicated on the following illustration.

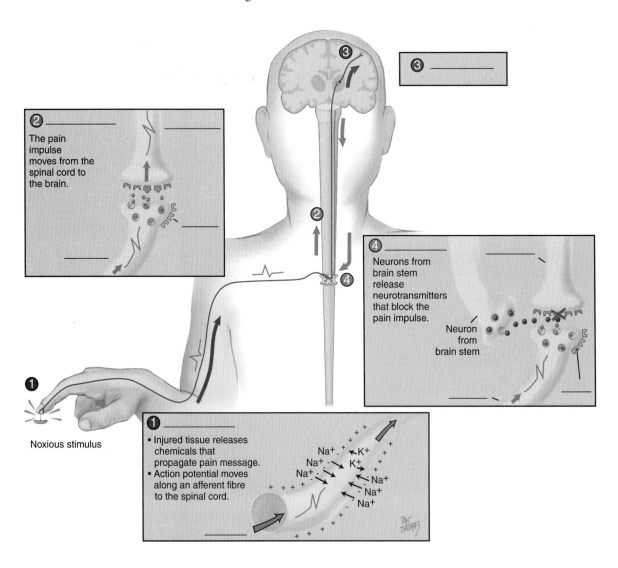

③ _____

② _____ _____

The pain impulse moves from the spinal cord to the brain.

④ _____

Neurons from brain stem release neurotransmitters that block the pain impulse.

Neuron from brain stem

① _____

Noxious stimulus

① _____

• Injured tissue releases chemicals that propagate pain message.
• Action potential moves along an afferent fibre to the spinal cord.

Na^+ K^+
Na^+ K^+
Na^+ Na^+
Na^+
Na^+

PAT THOMAS

REVIEW QUESTIONS

This test is for you to check your own mastery of the content. The answers are provided in Appendix A.

1. At what phase during nociception does the individual become aware of a painful sensation?

   a. modulation
   b. transduction
   c. perception
   d. transmission

2. While taking a history, the patient describes a burning, painful sensation that moves around his toes and bottoms of his feet. These symptoms are suggestive of:

   a. nociceptive pain.
   b. neuropathic pain.

3. During the physical examination, your patient is diaphoretic, pale, and complains of pain directly over the LUQ of the abdomen. This would be categorized as:

   a. cutaneous pain.
   b. somatic pain.
   c. visceral pain.
   d. psychogenic pain.

4. While caring for a preterm infant, you are aware that:

   a. inhibitory neurotransmitters are in sufficient supply by 15 weeks' gestation.
   b. the fetus has less capacity to feel pain.
   c. repetitive blood draws have minimal long-term consequences.
   d. the preterm infant is more sensitive to painful stimuli.

5. The most reliable indicator of pain in the adult is:

   a. degree of physical functioning.
   b. nonverbal behaviours.
   c. MRI findings.
   d. the patient's self-report.

6. While examining a broken arm of a four-year-old boy, select the appropriate assessment tool to evaluate his pain status.

   a. 0–10 numeric rating scale
   b. The Wong–Baker scale
   c. Simple descriptor scale
   d. 0–5 numeric rating scale

7. When a person presents with acute pain of the abdomen, following the initial examination, it is best to withhold analgesia until diagnostic testing is completed and a diagnosis is made.

   a. True
   b. False

8. For older adult postoperative patients, poorly controlled acute pain places them at higher risk for:

   a. atelectasis.
   b. increased myocardial oxygen demand.
   c. impaired wound healing.
   d. all of the above.

9. A 30-year-old female reports having persistent intense pain in her right arm related to trauma sustained from a car accident five months ago. She states that the slightest touch or clothing can exacerbate the pain. This report is suggestive of:

a. referred pain.
b. psychogenic pain.
c. Complex Regional Pain Syndrome.
d. cutaneous pain.

10. The PIPP is an appropriate pain assessment tool for:

a. cognitively impaired older adults.
b. children ages two to eight years.
c. infants.
d. premature infants.

11. A pain problem should be anticipated in a cognitively impaired older adult with a history of:

a. diabetes.
b. peripheral vascular disease.
c. COPD.
d. Parkinson's disease.

SKILLS LABORATORY/CLINICAL SETTING

You are now ready for the clinical component of the pain assessment. The purpose of the clinical component is to practise the examination on a peer in the skills laboratory or on a patient in the clinical setting and to achieve the following:

CLINICAL OBJECTIVES

1. Obtain an initial pain assessment on a classmate or patient.

2. Demonstrate a physical examination on a painful area and identify abnormal findings.

3. Select appropriate pain assessment tools for further follow-up and monitoring.

4. Record the history and physical examination findings accurately, assess the nature of the pain, and develop an appropriate plan of care.

Nutritional Assessment

PURPOSE

This chapter helps you to learn the components of nutritional assessment, including the assessment of dietary intake and nutritional status of individuals; to identify the possible occurrence, nature, and extent of impaired nutritional status (ranging from undernutrition to overnutrition), and to record the assessment accurately.

READING ASSIGNMENT

Jarvis, *Physical Examination and Health Assessment,* 1st Canadian ed., Chapter 11, pp. 195–219.

GLOSSARY

Study the following terms after completing the reading assignment. You should be able to cover the definition on the right and define the term out loud.

Android obesity ....excess body fat that is placed predominantly within the abdomen and upper body, as opposed to the hips and thighs

Anergy...a less-than-expected or absent immune reaction in response to the injection of antigens within the skin

Anthropometry ....measurement of the body, for example, height, weight, circumferences, skinfold thickness

Body mass index ....weight in kilograms divided by height in metres squared (W/H^2); value of 30 or more is indicative of obesity; value of less than 18.5 is indicative of undernutrition

Creatinine–height index (CHI) ....index or ratio sometimes used to assess body protein status

Daily reference intakes (DRIs) ....recommended amounts of nutrients to prevent deficiencies, reduce the risk of chronic disease, and avoid toxicity

Diet history ....a detailed record of dietary intake obtainable from 24-hour recalls, food frequency questionnaires, food diaries, and similar methods

Gynoid obesity ....excess body fat that is placed predominantly within the hips and thighs

Kwashiorkor.................................primarily a protein deficiency characterized by edema, growth failure, and muscle wasting

Malnutrition..............................may mean any nutrition disorder but usually refers to long-term nutritional inadequacies or excesses

Marasmic kwashiorkor..............combination of chronic energy deficit and chronic or acute protein deficiency

Marasmus...................................results from energy and protein deficiency, presenting with significant loss of body weight, skeletal muscle, and adipose tissue mass, but with serum protein concentrations relatively intact

Nitrogen balance........................condition in which nitrogen losses from the body are equal to nitrogen intake; the expected state of the healthy adult

Nutrition screening...................a process used to identify individuals at nutritional risk or with nutritional problems

Obesity..excessive accumulation of body fat; usually defined as 20% above desirable weight

Protein-calorie
malnutrition (PCM)..................inadequate consumption of protein and energy, resulting in a gradual body wasting and increased susceptibility to infection

Serum proteins...........................proteins present in serum that are indicators of the body's visceral protein status (for example: albumin, prealbumin, transferrin)

Waist-to-hip ratio (WHR).........waist or abdominal circumference divided by the hip or gluteal circumference; method for assessing fat distribution

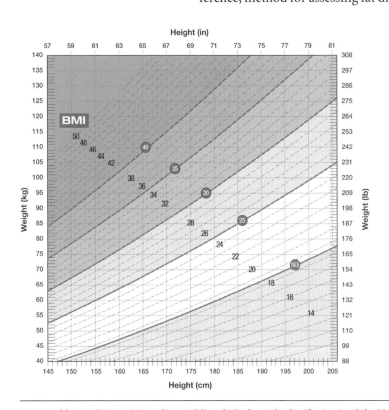

BMI interpretation for adults (World Health Organization (WHO, 2007):
    <18.5 Underweight
    18.5 to 24.9 Normal weight
    25.0 to 29.9 Overweight
    30.0 to 39.9 Obesity
    ≥40 Extreme obesity
    BMI interpretation for children ages 2 to 20 years (CDC, 2000):
    85th to 95th percentile = risk for overweight

From Health Canada. (2003). Canadian guidelines for body weight classification in adults (Catalogue No. H49-179/2003E; p. 37). Ottawa, ON: Health Canada. Retrieved June 6, 2008, from http://www.hc-sc.gc.ca/fn-an/alt_formats/hpfb-dgp-sa/pdf/nutrition/weight_book-livres_des_poids_e.pdf. Reproduced with the permission of the Minister of Public Works and Government Services Canada, 2008.

STUDY GUIDE

After completing the reading assignment, you should be able to answer the following questions in the spaces provided.

1. Define *nutritional status.*

2. Describe the unique nutritional needs for various developmental periods throughout the life cycle.

3. Describe the role cultural heritage and values may play in an individual's nutritional intake.

4. State three purposes of a nutritional assessment.

5. List and describe five factors that place an individual at nutritional risk.

6. Describe four sources of error that may occur when using the 24-hour diet recall.

7. Explain the clinical changes associated with each type of malnutrition:

Obesity _____

Marasmus _____

Kwashiorkor _____

Marasmus/kwashiorkor mix _____

REVIEW QUESTIONS

This test is for you to check your own mastery of the content. Answers are provided in Appendix A.

1. The balance between nutrient intake and nutrient requirements is described as:

   a. undernutrition.
   b. malnutrition.
   c. nutritional status.
   d. overnutrition.

2. To support the synthesis of maternal and fetal tissue during pregnancy, a weight gain of _____ is recommended.

   a. 11.5 to 16 kg
   b. 12.5 to 18 kg
   c. 7 to 11 kg
   d. Recommendation depends on BMI of mother at the start of the pregnancy.

3. All of the following are normal physiological changes in older adults that directly affect nutritional status, except:

   a. poor dentition
   b. decreased visual acuity
   c. increased gastrointestinal absorption
   d. diminished olfactory and taste sensitivity

4. Which of the following data would be obtained as part of a nutritional screening?

   a. temperature, pulse, and respiration
   b. blood pressure and genogram
   c. weight and nutrition intake history
   d. serum creatinine levels

5. Canada's Food Guide recommends that adults consume the following number of servings of grain products each day:

   a. 7–8 for females, and 8–10 for males
   b. 6–7 for females, and 8 for males
   c. 2 for females and males
   d. 2 for females, and 3 for males

6. The 24-hour recall of dietary intake:

   a. is an anthropometric measure of calories consumed.
   b. is a questionnaire or interview of everything eaten within the last 24 hours.
   c. is the same as a food frequency questionnaire.
   d. is a form of food diary.

7. The nutritional needs of a patient with trauma or major surgery:

   a. are met by fat reserves in obese individuals.
   b. may be two to three times greater than normal.
   c. can be met with intravenous fluids, supplemented with vitamins and electrolytes.
   d. are met by glycogen reserves.

8. Mary, a 15-year-old, has come for a school physical. During the interview, the examiner is told that menarche has not occurred. An explanation to be explored is:

    a. nutritional deficiency.
    b. alcohol intake.
    c. smoking history.
    d. possible elevated blood sugar.

9. Older adults are at risk for alteration in nutritional status. From the individuals described below, select the individual(s) who appear(s) least at risk.

    a. an 80-year-old widow who lives alone
    b. a 65-year-old widower who visits a senior centre with a meal program five days a week
    c. a 70-year-old with poor dentition who lives with a son
    d. a 73-year-old couple with low income and no transportation

10. Body weight as a percentage of ideal body weight is calculated to assess for malnutrition. Severe malnutrition is diagnosed when current body weight is:

    a. 80% to 90% of ideal weight.
    b. 70% to 80% of ideal weight.
    c. less than 70% of ideal body weight.
    d. 120% of ideal body weight.

11. The examiner is completing an initial assessment for a patient being admitted to a long-term care facility. The patient is unable to stand for a measurement of height. In order to obtain this important anthropometric information the examiner may:

    a. measure the waist-to-hip circumference.
    b. estimate the body mass index.
    c. measure arm span.
    d. obtain a mid-upper arm muscle circumference to estimate skeletal muscle reserve.

12. A skin testing or anergy panel has been ordered for a patient. This test is done to:

    a. determine serum protein levels.
    b. determine the need for adult immunization.
    c. assess for excessive exposure to ultraviolet light.
    d. assess for immunocompetence.

13. Which assessment finding indicates nutrition risk?

    a. BMI = 24
    b. serum albumin = 30 g/L
    c. current weight = 90 kg
    d. BMI = 19

14. Marasmus is often characterized by:

    a. severely depleted visceral proteins
    b. elevated triglycerides
    c. hyperglycemia
    d. low weight for height

15. Which BMI category in adults is indicative of obesity?

    a. 18.5–24.9
    b. 25.0–29.9
    c. 30.0–39.9
    d. <18.5

SKILLS LABORATORY/CLINICAL SETTING

You are now ready for the clinical component of the nutritional assessment. The purpose of the clinical component is to practise the steps of the assessment on a peer in the skills laboratory and to achieve the following:

CLINICAL OBJECTIVES

1. Identify persons at risk for developing malnutrition.

2. Develop an appreciation for cultural influences on nutritional status.

3. Use anthropometric measures and laboratory data to assess the nutritional status of an individual.

4. Use nutritional assessment in the provision of health care.

5. Record the assessment findings accurately.

INSTRUCTIONS

Practise the steps of the *Admission Nutrition Screening Tool* on a peer in the skills laboratory. This will familiarize you with the appropriate history and give you practice computing the derived weight measures. Likely you will not have access to a peer's serum laboratory data; however, the history and physical examination data will give you all the data you need to make a clinical judgement on a well adult. Record your findings using one of the Assessment Forms that follow.

Finally, review the questions in the "Determine Your Nutritional Health" checklist with an aging adult. This is a three-step approach for nutrition screening of older adults. The nutrition checklist is completed by the older person or caregiver and identifies major risk factors and indicators of poor nutritional status.

NOTES

Jarvis, Luctkar-Flude: PHYSICAL EXAMINATION AND HEALTH ASSESSMENT, First Canadian Edition,
Student Laboratory Manual. Copyright © 2009 by Elsevier Canada, a division of Reed Elsevier Canada, Ltd. All rights reserved.

Admission Nutrition Screening Tool

A. DIAGNOSIS

If the patient has at least ONE of the following diagnoses, circle and proceed to section E to consider the patient
AT NUTRITIONAL RISK and stop here.

- Anorexia nervosa/bulimia nervosa
- Malabsorption (celiac sprue, ulcerative colitis, Crohn's disease, short bowel syndrome)
- Multiple trauma (closed-head injury, penetrating trauma, multiple fractures)
- Decubitus ulcers
- Major gastrointestinal surgery within the past year
- Cachexia (temporal wasting, muscle wasting, cancer, cardiac)
- Coma
- Diabetes
- End-stage liver disease
- End-stage renal disease
- Nonhealing wounds

B. NUTRITION INTAKE HISTORY

If the patient has at least ONE of the following symptoms, circle and proceed to section E to consider the patient
AT NUTRITIONAL RISK and stop here.

- Diarrhea ($>$500 mL $\times$ 2 days)
- Vomiting ($>$5 days)
- Reduced intake ($<$1/2 normal intake for $>$5 days)

C. AVERAGE BODY WEIGHT STANDARDS (BMI)

Determine the patient's current BMI by measuring their height and weight and compare it to the WHO standards for average weight. (Refer to
p. 74 of the lab manual, and pp. 152 and 207 of the text.)

If their BMI is $<$18.5, proceed to section E to consider the patient AT NUTRITIONAL RISK and stop here.

D. WEIGHT HISTORY

Any recent unplanned weight loss? No ___ Yes ___ Amount (lb or kg) ___
    If yes, within the past ___ weeks or ___ months
    Current weight (lb or kg) ___
    Usual weight (lb of kg) ___
    Height (ft, in, or cm) ___

Find percentage of weight lost: $\dfrac{\text{usual wt} - \text{current wt}}{\text{usual wt}} \times 100 = $ _____ % wt loss

Compare the % wt loss with the chart values and circle appropriate value:

LENGTH OF TIME	SIGNIFICANT (%)	SEVERE (%)
1 week	1–2	$>$2
2–3 weeks	2–3	$>$3
1 months	4–5	$>$5
3 months	7–8	$>$8
5+ months	10	$>$10

If the patient has experienced a significant or severe weight loss, proceed to section E and consider the patient AT NUTRITIONAL RISK.

E. NURSE ASSESSMENT

Using the above criteria, what is this patient's nutritional risk? (circle one)

    LOW NUTRITIONAL RISK

    AT NUTRITIONAL RISK

Nutrition Risk Classification: A Reproductive & Valid Tool for Nurses (Table 1—Admission Nutrition Screening Tool) by Debra S.
Kovacevich, et al. In *Nutrition in Clinical Practice* (February 1997) 12:20–25.

NOTES

The warning signs of poor nutritional health are often overlooked. Use this checklist to find out if you or someone you know is at nutritional risk.

DETERMINE YOUR NUTRITIONAL HEALTH

Read the statements below. Circle the number in the yes column for those that apply to you or someone you know. For each yes answer, score the number in the box. Total your nutritional score.

	YES
I have an illness or condition that made me change the kind and/or amount of food I eat.	2
I eat fewer than 2 meals per day.	3
I eat few fruits or vegetables, or milk products.	2
I have 3 or more drinks of beer, liquor or wine almost every day.	2
I have tooth or mouth problems that make it hard for me to eat.	2
I don't always have enough money to buy the food I need.	4
I eat alone most of the time.	1
I take 3 or more different prescribed or over-the-counter drugs a day.	1
Without wanting to, I have lost or gained 4.5 kg in the last 6 months.	2
I am not always physically able to shop, cook, and/or feed myself.	2
	TOTAL

Total Your Nutritional Score. If it's —

0-2 Good! Recheck your nutritional score in 6 months.

3-5 You are at moderate nutritional risk. See what can be done to improve your eating habits and lifestyle. Your office on aging, senior nutrition program, senior citizens centre, or health department can help. Recheck your nutritional score in 3 months.

6 or more You are at high nutritional risk. Bring this checklist the next time you see your doctor, dietitian, or other qualified health or social service professional. Talk with them about any problems you may have. Ask for help to improve your nutritional health.

These materials developed and distributed by the Nutrition Screening Initiative, a project of:

 AMERICAN ACADEMY OF FAMILY PHYSICIANS

 THE AMERICAN DIETETIC ASSOCIATION

 NATIONAL COUNCIL ON THE AGING, INC.

* Remember that warning signs suggest risk but do not represent diagnosis of any condition.

Features of the Scored Patient-Generated Subjective Global Assessment (PG-SGA)

(Select appropriate category with a checkmark, or enter numerical value where indicated by "#".)

A. History

1. Weight change

   Overall loss in past 6 months: amount = # _____ kg; % loss = # _____

   Change in past 2 weeks: _____ increase, _____ no change, _____ decrease

2. Dietary intake change (relative to normal)

   ___ No change

   ___ Change _____ duration = # _____ weeks

   ___ Type: _____ suboptimal solid diet _____ full liquid diet _____ hypocaloric liquids

   ___ starvation

3. Gastrointestinal symptoms (that persisted for >2 weeks)

   ___ none _____ nausea _____ vomiting

   ___ diarrhea _____ anorexia

4. Functional capacity

   ___ No dysfunction (e.g., full capacity)

   ___ Dysfunction _____ duration = # _____ weeks

   ___ Type: _____ working suboptimally _____ ambulatory _____ bedridden

5. Disease and its relation to nutritional requirements

   Primary diagnosis (specify)

   Metabolic demand (stress): _____ no stress _____ low stress _____ moderate stress
   _____ high stress

B. Physical (FOR EACH TRAIT SPECIFY 0 = NORMAL, 1+ = MILD, 2+ = MODERATE, 3+ = SEVERE)

   # ___ loss of subcutaneous fat (triceps, chest)

   # ___ muscle wasting (quadriceps, deltoids)

   # ___ ankle edema

   # ___ sacral edema

   # ___ ascites

C. SGA rating (SELECT ONE)

   ___ A = Well nourished

   ___ B = Moderately malnourished (or suspected of being malnourished)

   ___ C = Severely malnourished

Reprinted with permission from Detsky AJ, McLaughlin JR, Baker JP, et al. What is subjective global assessment of nutritional status? *J Parenter Enteral Nutr.* 1987;11:9.

UNIT 3

Physical Examination

Chapter Twelve

Skin, Hair, and Nails

PURPOSE

This chapter helps you to learn the structure and function of the skin and its appendages; to understand the rationale for and the methods of inspection and palpation of the skin; and to record the assessment accurately.

READING ASSIGNMENT

Jarvis, *Physical Examination and Health Assessment*, 1st Canadian ed., Chapter 12, pp. 221–269.

GLOSSARY

Study the following terms after completing the reading assignment. You should be able to cover the definition on the right and define the term out loud.

Alopecia.......................................(baldness) hair loss

Annular ....circular shape to skin lesion

Bulla...elevated cavity containing free fluid, >1 cm diameter

Confluent ....skin lesions that run together

Crust ....thick, dried-out exudate left on skin when vesicles/pustules burst or dry up

Cyanosis ....dusky blue colour to skin or mucous membranes due to increased amount of unoxygenated hemoglobin

Erosion ....scooped out, shallow depression in skin

Erythema....................................intense redness of the skin due to excess blood in dilated superficial capillaries, as in fever or inflammation

Excoriation ....self-inflicted abrasion on skin due to scratching

Fissure ....linear crack in skin extending into dermis

Furuncle ....(boil) suppurative inflammatory skin lesion due to infected hair follicle

Hemangioma ....skin lesion due to benign proliferation of blood vessels in the dermis

Iris...target shape of skin lesion

Jaundice....................................yellow colour to skin, palate, and sclera due to excess bilirubin in the blood

Keloid ....hypertrophic scar, elevated beyond site of original injury

Lichenification ....tightly packed set of papules that thickens skin, from prolonged intense scratching

Lipoma ....benign fatty tumour

Maceration................................softening of tissue by soaking

Macule ....flat skin lesion with only a colour change

Nevus ....(mole) circumscribed skin lesion due to excess melanocytes

Nodule ....elevated skin lesion, >1 cm diameter

Pallor ....excessively pale, whitish-pink colour to lightly pigmented skin

Papule...palpable skin lesion of <1 cm diameter

Plaque...skin lesion in which papules coalesce or come together

Pruritus......................................itching

Purpura......................................red-purple skin lesion due to blood in tissues from breaks in blood vessels

Pustule..elevated cavity containing thick turbid fluid

Scale ....compact desiccated flakes of skin from shedding of dead skin cells

Telangiectasia ....skin lesion due to permanently enlarged and dilated blood vessels that are visible

Ulcer...sloughing of necrotic inflammatory tissue that causes a deep depression in skin, extending into dermis

Vesicle ....elevated cavity containing free fluid up to 1 cm diameter

Wheal..raised red skin lesion due to interstitial fluid

Zosteriform................................linear shape of skin lesion along a nerve route

STUDY GUIDE

After completing the reading assignment, you should be able to answer the following questions in the spaces provided.

1. List the three layers associated with the skin, and describe the contents of each layer.

2. Define two types of human hair.

3. Differentiate between sebaceous, eccrine, and apocrine glands.

4. List at least five functions of the skin.

5. List at least six variables that are external to the skin itself that can influence skin colour.

6. Describe the appearance of pallor, erythema, cyanosis, and jaundice, both in light-skinned and in dark-skinned persons. State common causes of each.

7. List causes of changes in skin temperature, texture, moisture, mobility, and turgor.

8. Describe each grade on the four-point grading scale for pitting edema.

9. Distinguish the terms *primary* versus *secondary* in reference to skin lesions.

10. The white linear markings that normally are visible through the nail and on the pink nail bed are

    termed _____.

11. Describe the following findings that are common variations on the infant's skin:

    Mongolian spot _____

    Café au lait spot _____

    Erythema toxicum _____

    Cutis marmorata _____

    Physiological jaundice _____

    Milia _____

12. Describe the following findings that are common variations on the older adult's skin:

    Lentigines _____

    Seborrheic keratosis _____

    Actinic keratosis _____

    Acrochordons (skin tags) _____

    Sebaceous hyperplasia _____

13. Differentiate between these purpuric lesions: petechiae; ecchymosis; hematoma.

14. Differentiate between the appearance of the skin rash of these childhood illnesses: measles (rubeola); German measles (rubella); chickenpox (varicella).

15. List and describe three skin lesions associated with AIDS.

16. Contrast a furuncle with an abscess.

17. Describe the appearance of these conditions of the nails: koilonychia; paronychia; Beau's line; splinter hemorrhages; onycholysis; clubbing.

18. Define and give an example of the following primary skin lesions: macule; papule; plaque; nodule; tumour; wheal; vesicle; pustule.

And of these secondary lesions: crust; scale; fissure; erosion; ulcer; excoriation; scar; atrophic scar; lichenification; keloid.

Fill in the labels indicated on the following illustrations.

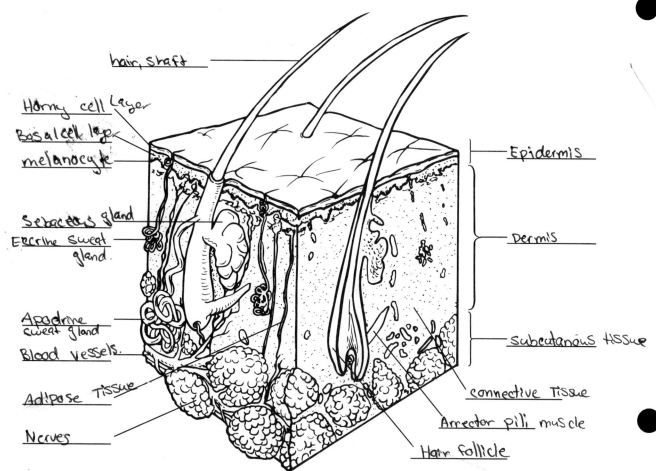

hair, shaft

Horny cell Layer

Basal cell layer

melanocyte

Sebaceous gland

Eccrine sweat gland.

Apocrine sweat gland

Blood vessels.

Adipose Tissue

Nerves

Epidermis

Dermis

Subcutaneous tissue

connective Tissue

Arrector pili muscle

Hair follicle

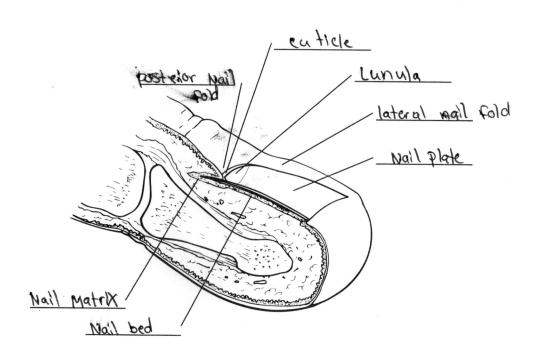

cuticle

Lunula

lateral nail fold

Nail plate

Posterior Nail fold

Nail Matrix

Nail bed

REVIEW QUESTIONS

This test is for you to check your own mastery of the content. Answers are provided in Appendix A.

1. Select the best description of the secretion of the eccrine glands.

   a. thick, milky
   b. dilute saline solution
   c. protective lipid substance
   d. keratin

2. Nevus is the medical term for:

   a. a freckle.
   b. a birthmark.
   c. an infected hair follicle.
   d. a mole.

3. To assess for early jaundice, you will assess:

   a. sclera and hard palate.
   b. nail beds.
   c. lips.
   d. all visible skin surfaces.

4. Checking for skin temperature is best accomplished by using:

   a. palmar surface of the hands.
   b. ventral surface of the hands.
   c. fingertips.
   d. dorsal surface of the hands.

5. Skin turgor is assessed by picking up a large fold of skin on the anterior chest under the clavicle. This is done to determine the presence of:

   a. edema.
   b. dehydration.
   c. vitiligo.
   d. scleroderma.

6. You note a lesion during an examination. Select the description that is most complete.

   a. raised, irregular lesion the size of a quarter, located on dorsum of left hand
   b. open lesion with no drainage or odour approximately 1/4 inch in diameter
   c. pedunculated lesion below left scapula with consistent red colour, no drainage or odour
   d. dark brown, raised lesion, with irregular border, on dorsum of right foot, 3 cm in size with no drainage

7. You examine nail beds for clubbing. The normal angle between the nail base and the nails is:

   a. 60 degrees.
   b. 100 degrees.
   c. 160 degrees.
   d. 180 degrees.

8. The capillary beds should refill after being depressed in:

   a. <1 second.
   b. >2 seconds.
   c. 1–2 seconds.
   d. time is not significant as long as colour returns.

9. During a routine visit, M.B., age 78 years, asks about small, round, flat, brown macules on the hands. Your best response after examining the areas is:

   a. "These are the result of sun exposure and do not require treatment."
   b. "These are related to exposure to the sun. They may become cancerous."
   c. "These are the skin tags that occur with aging. No treatment is required."
   d. "I'm glad you brought this to my attention. I will arrange for a biopsy."

10. An area of thin, shiny skin with decreased visibility of normal skin markings is called:

    a. lichenification.
    b. plaque.
    c. atrophy.
    d. keloid.

11. Flattening of the angle between the nail and its base is:

    a. found in subacute bacterial endocarditis.
    b. a description of spoon-shaped nails.
    c. related to calcium deficiency.
    d. described as clubbing.

12. The configuration for individual lesions arranged in circles or arcs, as occurs with ringworm, is called:

    a. linear.
    b. clustered.
    c. annular.
    d. gyrate.

13. The "A" in the ABCDE rule stands for:

    a. accuracy.
    b. appearance.
    c. asymmetry.
    d. attenuated.

14. A risk factor for melanoma is:

    a. brown eyes.
    b. darkly pigmented skin.
    c. skin that freckles or burns before tanning.
    d. use of sunscreen products.

Match column A to column B—items in column B may be used more than once.

Column A—Descriptor

15. ____ basal cell layer
16. ____ aids protection by cushioning
17. ____ collagen
18. ____ adipose tissue
19. ____ uniformly thin
20. ____ stratum corneum
21. ____ elastic tissue

Column B—Skin Layer

a. epidermis
b. dermis
c. subcutaneous layer

Column A—Descriptor

22. ____ pallor
23. ____ erythema
24. ____ cyanosis
25. ____ jaundice

Column B—Colour Change

a. intense redness of the skin due to excess blood in the dilated superficial capillaries
b. bluish mottled colour that signifies decreased perfusion
c. absence of red-pink tones from the oxygenated hemoglobin in blood
d. increase in bilirubin in the blood causing a yellow colour in the skin

Column A—Descriptor

Column B—Skin Colour Change

26. ____ tiny, punctate red macules and papules on the cheeks, trunk, chest, back, and buttocks

a. harlequin

27. ____ lower half of body turns red, upper half blanches

b. erythema toxicum

28. ____ transient mottling on trunk and extremities

c. acrocyanosis

29. ____ bluish colour around the lips, hands, and fingernails, pigmentation, and feet and toenails

d. physiological jaundice

30. ____ large round or oval patch of light brown usually present at birth

e. carotenemia

f. café au lait

31. ____ yellowing of skin, sclera, and mucous membranes due to increased numbers of red blood cells hemolyzed following birth

g. cutis marmorata

32. ____ yellow-orange colour in light-skinned persons from large amounts of foods containing carotene

SKILLS LABORATORY/CLINICAL SETTING

You are now ready for the clinical component of the integumentary system. Usually the clinical examination of the integumentary system is performed along with the examination of each particular body region. The purpose of practising the steps of this examination separately is so that you begin to think of the skin and its appendages as a separate organ system, and so that you learn the components of skin examination.

CLINICAL OBJECTIVES

1. Inspect and palpate the skin, noting its colour, vascularity, edema, moisture, temperature, texture, thickness, mobility and turgor, and any lesions.

2. Inspect the fingernails, noting colour, shape, and any lesions.

3. Inspect the hair, noting texture, distribution, and any lesions.

4. Record the history and physical examination findings accurately, reach an assessment of the health state, and develop a plan of care.

INSTRUCTIONS

Prepare the examination setting. Wash your hands. Practise the steps of the examination on a peer in the skills laboratory, giving appropriate instructions as you proceed. Choosing a peer from an ethnic background other than your own will further heighten your recognition of the range of normal skin tones. Record your findings using the regional write-up sheet that follows. The front of the page is intended as a worksheet; the back of the page is intended for your narrative summary recording using the SOAP format.

Note the student performance checklist that follows the regional write-up sheet. It lists the essential behaviours you should display as an examiner, and it may be used by your clinical instructor to evaluate your clinical teaching of the skin self-examination.

NOTES

REGIONAL WRITE-UP—SKIN, HAIR, AND NAILS

Date _____

Examiner _____

Patient _____ Age _____ Gender _____

Occupation _____

I. Health History

	No	Yes, explain
1. Any previous **skin disease**?		
2. Any change in skin colour or **pigmentation**?		
3. Any changes in a **mole**?		
4. Excessive **dryness** or **moisture**?		
5. Any skin **itching**?		
6. Any excess **bruising**?		
7. Any skin **rash** or **lesions**?		
8. Taking any **medications**?		
9. Any recent hair loss?		
10. Any change in nails?		
11. Any environmental hazards for skin?		
12. How do you take care of skin? Sunscreen?		

II. Physical Examination

A. Inspect and palpate skin

Colour _____

Pigmentation _____

Temperature _____

Moisture _____

Texture _____

Thickness _____

Any edema _____

Mobility and turgor _____

Vascularity and bruising _____

Any lesions (describe) _____

B. Inspect and palpate hair

Colour _____

Texture _____

Distribution _____

Any lesions (describe) _____

C. Inspect and palpate nails

Shape and contour _____

Consistency _____

Distribution _____

Colour _____

Capillary refill _____

D. Teach skin self-examination

REGIONAL WRITE-UP—SKIN, HAIR, AND NAILS

Summarize your findings using the SOAP format.

Subjective (Reason for seeking care, health history)

Objective (Physical examination findings)

Record distribution of any rash or lesions below

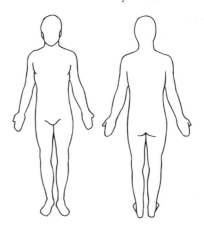

Assessment (Assessment of problem, diagnosis)

Plan (Diagnostic evaluation, follow-up care, teaching)

STUDENT COMPETENCY CHECKLIST

TEACHING SKIN SELF-EXAMINATION (SSE)

	S	U	Comments
I. Cognitive			
1. Explain:			
a. Why skin is examined			
b. Who should perform skin self-examination			
c. Frequency of skin examination			
2. Define the ABCDE rule			
3. Describe any equipment the patient may need			
II. Performance			
1. Explains to patient need for SSE			
2. Instructs patient on technique of SSE by:			
a. demonstrating the order and body positioning for inspecting skin			
b. describing normal skin characteristics			
c. describing abnormal findings to look for			
3. Instructs patient to report unusual findings to nurse or physician at once			

NOTES

Head, Face, and Neck, Including Regional Lymphatics

PURPOSE

This chapter helps you to learn the location and function of structures in the head and neck; to learn to perform inspection and palpation of the head and neck; and to record the assessment accurately.

READING ASSIGNMENT

Jarvis, *Physical Examination and Health Assessment,* 1st Canadian ed., Chapter 13, pp. 271–296.

AUDIO-VISUAL ASSIGNMENT

Jarvis, *Physical Examination and Health Assessment DVD Series: Head, Eyes, and Ears*

GLOSSARY

Study the following terms after completing the reading assignment. You should be able to cover the definition on the right and define the term out loud.

Bruit...........................blowing, swooshing sound heard through the stethoscope over an area of abnormal blood flow

Dysphagia ....difficulty in swallowing

Goiter...........................increase in size of thyroid gland that occurs with hyperthyroidism

Lymphadenopathy ....enlargement of the lymph nodes due to infection, allergy, or neoplasm

Macrocephalic ....abnormally large head

Microcephalic...........................abnormally small head

Normocephalic..........................round symmetric skull that is appropriately related to body size

Torticollis..................................head tilt due to shortening or spasm of one sternomastoid muscle

Vertigo ....illusory sensation of either the room or one's own body spinning; it is not the same as dizziness

STUDY GUIDE

After completing the reading assignment and the audio-visual assignment, you should be able to answer the following questions in the spaces provided.

1. The major neck muscles are the _____.

2. Name the borders of two regions in the neck, the anterior triangle, and the posterior triangle.

3. List the facial structures that should appear symmetric when inspecting the head.

4. Describe the characteristics of lymph nodes often associated with:

   Acute infection

   Chronic inflammation

   Cancer

5. Differentiate *caput succedaneum* from *cephalhematoma* in the newborn infant.

6. Describe the tonic neck reflex in the infant.

7. Describe the characteristics of normal cervical lymph nodes during childhood.

8. List the condition(s) associated with parotid gland enlargement.

9. Describe the facial characteristics that occur with Down syndrome.

10. Contrast the facial characteristics of hyperthyroidism versus hypothyroidism.

Fill in the labels indicated on the following illustrations.

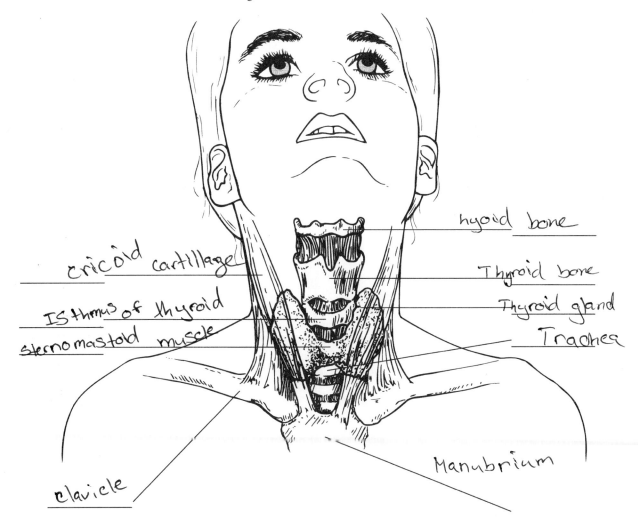

hyoid bone

cricoid cartillage

Thyroid bone

Isthmus of thyroid

Thyroid gland

sternomastoid muscle

Trachea

Manubrium

clavicle

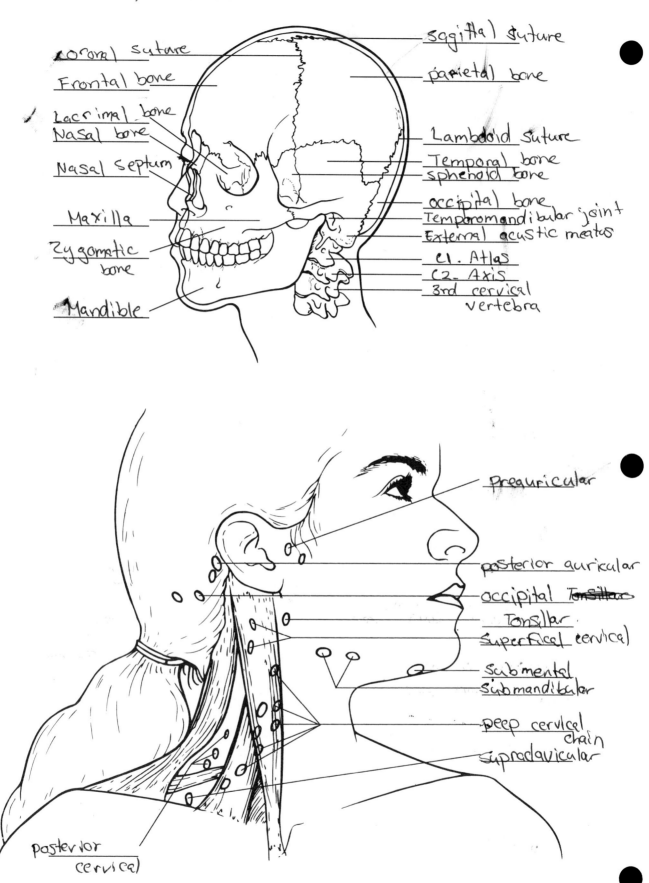

Coronal suture
Frontal bone
Lacrimal bone
Nasal bone
Nasal septum
Maxilla
Zygomatic bone
Mandible

Sagittal suture
parietal bone
Lambdoid suture
Temporal bone
Sphenoid bone
occipital bone
Temporomandibular joint
External acustic meatus
C1. Atlas
C2. Axis
3rd cervical vertebra

Preauricular
posterior auricular
occipital ~~Tonsillar~~
Tonsilar
Superficial cervical
Submental
Submandibular
Deep cervical chain
Supraclavicular

posterior cervical

Jarvis, Luctkar-Flude: PHYSICAL EXAMINATION AND HEALTH ASSESSMENT, First Canadian Edition,
Student Laboratory Manual. Copyright © 2009 by Elsevier Canada, a division of Reed Elsevier Canada, Ltd. All rights reserved.

REVIEW QUESTIONS

This test is for you to check your own mastery of the content. Answers are provided in Appendix A.

1. Identify the facial bone that articulates at a joint instead of a suture.

   a. zygomatic
   b. maxilla
   c. nasal
   d. mandible

2. Identify the blood vessel that runs diagonally across the sternomastoid muscle.

   a. temporal artery
   b. carotid artery
   c. external jugular vein
   d. internal jugular vein

3. The isthmus of the thyroid gland lies just below the:

   a. mandible.
   b. cricoid cartilage.
   c. hyoid cartilage.
   d. thyroid cartilage.

4. Select the statement that is true regarding cluster headaches.

   a. May be precipitated by alcohol and daytime napping.
   b. Usual occurrence is two per month, each lasting one to three days.
   c. Characterized as throbbing.
   d. Tend to be supraorbital, retro-orbital, or frontotemporal.

5. Select the symptom that is least likely to indicate a possible malignancy.

   a. history of radiation therapy to head, neck, or upper chest
   b. history of using chewing tobacco
   c. history of large alcohol consumption
   d. tenderness

6. Providing resistance while the patient shrugs the shoulders is a test of the status of cranial nerve:

   a. II.
   b. V.
   c. IX.
   d. XI.

7. Upon examination, the fontanels should feel:

   a. tense or bulging.
   b. depressed or sunken.
   c. firm, slightly concave, and well defined.
   d. pulsating.

8. If the thyroid gland is enlarged bilaterally, which of the following manoeuvres is appropriate?

   a. Check for deviation of the trachea.
   b. Listen for a bruit over the carotid arteries.
   c. Listen for a murmur over the aortic area.
   d. Listen for a bruit over the thyroid lobes.

9. It is normal to palpate a few lymph nodes in the neck of a healthy person. What are the characteristics of these nodes?

   a. mobile, soft, nontender
   b. large, clumped, tender
   c. matted, fixed, tender, hard
   d. matted, fixed, nontender

10. Cephalhematoma is associated with:

   a. subperiosteal hemorrhage.
   b. craniotabes.
   c. bossing.
   d. congenital syphilis.

11. Normal cervical lymph nodes are:

    a. smaller than 1 cm.
    b. warm to palpation.
    c. fixed.
    d. firm.

12. A throbbing, unilateral pain associated with nausea, vomiting, and photophobia is characteristic of:

    a. cluster headache.
    b. subarachnoid hemorrhage.
    c. migraine headache.
    d. tension headache.

Match column A with column B.

Column A—Lymph Nodes	Column B—Location
13. _____ Preauricular	a. above and behind the clavicle
14. _____ Posterior auricular	b. deep under the sternomastoid muscle
15. _____ Occipital	c. in front of the ear
16. _____ Submental	d. in the posterior triangle along the edge of the trapezius muscle
17. _____ Submandibular	e. superficial to the mastoid process
18. _____ Jugulodigastric	f. at the base of the skull
19. _____ Superficial cervical	g. halfway between the angle and the tip of the mandible
20. _____ Deep cervical	h. behind the tip of the mandible
21. _____ Posterior cervical	i. under the angle of the mandible
22. _____ Supraclavicular	j. overlying the sternomastoid muscle

SKILLS LABORATORY/CLINICAL SETTINGS

You are now ready for the clinical component of the head, face, and neck chapter. The purpose of the clinical component is to practise the steps of the head, face, and neck examination on a peer in the skills laboratory and to achieve the following objectives:

CLINICAL OBJECTIVES

1. Collect a health history related to pertinent signs and symptoms of the head and neck.

2. Inspect and palpate the skull, noting size, contour, lumps, or tenderness.

3. Inspect the face, noting facial expression, symmetry, skin characteristics, or lesions.

4. Inspect and palpate the neck for symmetry, range of motion, and integrity of lymph nodes, trachea, and thyroid gland.

5. Record the findings systematically, reach an assessment of the health state, and develop a plan of care.

INSTRUCTIONS

Prepare the examination setting. Wash your hands. Practise the steps of the examination on a peer in the skills laboratory, giving appropriate instructions as you proceed. Record your findings using the regional write-up sheet that follows. The front of the page is intended as a worksheet; the back of the page is intended for your narrative summary recording using the SOAP format.

NOTES

NOTES

REGIONAL WRITE-UP—HEAD, FACE, AND NECK

Date _____

Examiner _____

Patient _____ Age _____ Gender _____

Occupation _____

I. Health History

	No	Yes, explain
1. Any unusually frequent or unusually severe **headaches**?		
2. Any **head injury**?		
3. Experienced any **dizziness**?		
4. Any neck **pain**?		
5. Any **lumps** or **swelling** in head or neck?		
6. Any surgery on head or neck?		

II. Physical Examination

A. Inspect and palpate the skull

General size and contour _____

Deformities, lumps, tenderness _____

Temporal artery _____

Temporomandibular joint _____

B. Inspect the face

Facial expression _____

Symmetry of structures _____

Involuntary movements _____

Edema _____

Masses or lesions _____

Colour and texture of skin _____

C. Inspect the neck

Symmetry _____

Range of motion, active _____

Test strength of cervical muscles _____

Abnormal pulsations _____

Enlargement of thyroid _____

Enlargement of lymph and salivary glands _____

D. Palpate the lymph nodes

Exact location _____

Size and shape _____

Presence or absence of tenderness _____

Freely movable, adherent to deeper structures, or matted together _____

Presence of surrounding inflammation _____

Texture (hard, soft, firm) _____

E. Palpate the trachea

F. Palpate the thyroid gland

G. Auscultate the thyroid gland (if enlarged)

REGIONAL WRITE-UP—HEAD, FACE, AND NECK

Summarize your findings using the SOAP format.

Subjective (Reason for seeking care, health history)

Objective (Physical examination findings)

Assessment (Assessment of health state or problem, diagnosis)

Plan (Diagnostic evaluation, follow-up care, patient teaching)

Eyes

PURPOSE

This chapter helps you to learn the structure and function of the external and internal components of the eyes; to learn the methods of examination of vision, external eye, and ocular fundus; and to record the assessment accurately.

READING ASSIGNMENT

Jarvis, *Physical Examination and Health Assessment,* 1st Canadian ed., Chapter 14, pp. 297–340.

AUDIO-VISUAL ASSIGNMENT

Jarvis, *Physical Examination and Health Assessment DVD Series: Head, Eyes, and Ears*

GLOSSARY

Study the following terms after completing the reading assignment. You should be able to cover the definition on the right and define the term out loud.

Accommodation ....adaptation of the eye for near vision by increasing the curvature of the lens

Anisocoria ....unequal pupil size

Arcus senilis ....grey-white arc or circle around the limbus of the iris that is common with aging

Argyll Robertson pupil ....pupil does not react to light; does constrict with accommodation

Astigmatism ....refractive error of vision due to differences in curvature in refractive surfaces of the eye (cornea and lens)

A-V crossing ....crossing paths of an artery and vein in the ocular fundus

Bitemporal hemianopsia ....loss of both temporal visual fields

Blepharitis ....inflammation of the glands and eyelash follicles along the margin of the eyelids

Cataract ....opacity of the lens of the eye that develops slowly with aging and gradu-ally obstructs vision

Chalazion ....infection or retention cyst of a meibomian gland, showing as a beady nodule on the eyelid

Conjunctivitis...........................infection of the conjunctiva, "pinkeye"

Cotton-wool area........................abnormal soft exudates visible as grey-white areas on the ocular fundus

Cup-disc ratio ....ratio of the width of the physiological cup to the width of the optic disc, normally half or less

Diopter ....unit of strength of the lens settings on the ophthalmoscope that changes focus on the eye structures

Diplopia ....double vision

Drusen..benign deposits on the ocular fundus that show as round yellow dots and occur commonly with aging

Ectropion ....lower eyelid loose and rolling outward

Entropion...................................lower eyelid rolling inward

Exophthalmos ....protruding eyeballs

Fovea..area of keenest vision at the centre of the macula on the ocular fundus

Glaucoma ....a group of eye diseases characterized by increased intraocular pressure

Hordeolum.................................(stye) red, painful pustule that is a localized infection of hair follicle at eyelid margin

Lid lag ....the abnormal white rim of sclera visible between the upper eyelid and the iris when a person moves the eyes downward

Macula ....round darker area of the ocular fundus that mediates vision only from the central visual field

Microaneurysm..........................abnormal finding of round red dots on the ocular fundus that are local-ized dilations of small vessels

Miosis ....constricted pupils

Mydriasis...................................dilated pupils

Myopia......................................."nearsighted"; refractive error in which near vision is better than far vision

Nystagmus..................................involuntary, rapid, rhythmic movement of the eyeball

OD..oculus dexter, or right eye

Optic atrophy.............................pallor of the optic disc due to partial or complete death of optic nerve

Optic disc...................................area of ocular fundus in which blood vessels exit and enter

OS..oculus sinister, or left eye

Papilledema ....stasis of blood flow out of the ocular fundus; sign of increased intracra-nial pressure

Presbyopia..................................decrease in power of accommodation that occurs with aging

Pterygium ....triangular opaque tissue on the nasal side of the conjunctiva that grows toward the centre of the cornea

Ptosis ....drooping of upper eyelid over the iris and possibly covering pupil

Red reflex ....red glow that appears to fill the person's pupil when first visualized through the ophthalmoscope

Strabismus ....(squint, crossed eye) disparity of the eye axes

Xanthelasma...............................soft, raised yellow plaques occurring on the skin at the inner corners of the eyes

STUDY GUIDE

After completing the reading assignment and the audio-visual assignment, you should be able to answer the following questions in the spaces provided.

1. Name the six sets of extraocular muscles and the cranial nerve that innervates each one.

2. Name and describe the three concentric coats of the eyeball.

3. Name the functions of the ciliary body, the pupil, and the iris.

4. Describe the anterior chamber, posterior chamber, and the vitreous body.

5. Describe how an image formed on the retina compares with an object's actual appearance in the outside world.

6. Describe the lacrimal system.

7. Define pupillary light reflex, fixation, and accommodation.

8. Concerning the pupillary light reflex, describe and contrast a direct light reflex with a consensual light reflex.

9. Identify common age-related changes in the eye.

10. Discuss the most common causes of decreased visual function in the older adult.

11. Explain the statement that normal visual acuity is 20/20.

12. Describe the method of testing for presbyopia.

13. To test for accommodation, the person focuses on a distant object, then shifts the gaze to a near object about six inches away. At near distance, you would expect the pupils to _____ (dilate/costrict), and the axes of the eyes to _____.

14. Concerning malalignment of the eye axes, contrast phoria with tropia.

15. Describe abnormal findings of tissue colour that are possible on the conjunctiva and sclera, and their significance.

16. Describe the method of everting the upper eyelid for examination.

17. Contrast *pingueculae* with *pterygium*.

18. Contrast the use of the negative diopter or red lens settings with the positive diopter or black lens settings on the ophthalmoscope.

19. Explain the rationale for testing for strabismus during early childhood.

20. Describe these findings and explain their significance: epicanthal fold; pseudostrabismus; ophthalmia neonatorum; Brushfield's spots.

21. Describe the following four types of "red eye" and explain their significance:

   a. Conjunctivitis:

   b. Subconjunctival hemorrhage:

   c. Iritis:

   d. Acute glaucoma:

Fill in the labels indicated on the following illustrations.

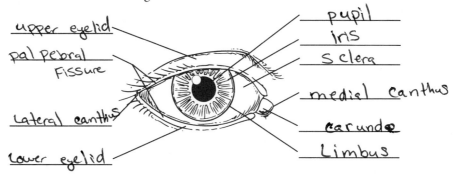

upper eyelid

palpebral Fissure

Lateral canthus

lower eyelid

pupil

iris

sclera

mediel canthus

carunde

Limbus

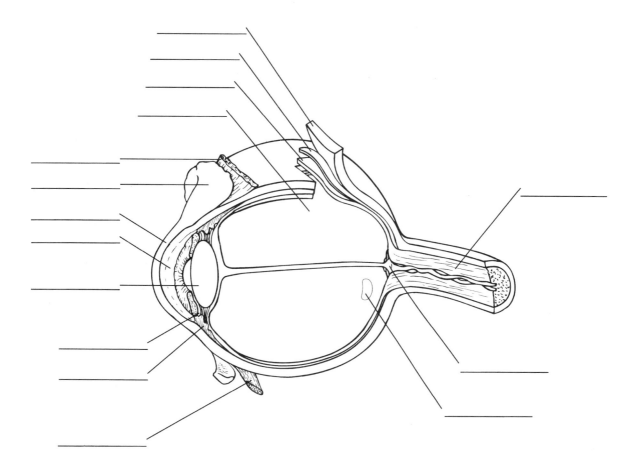

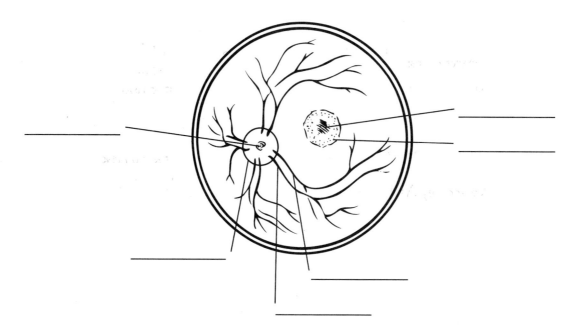

This test is for you to check your own mastery of the content. Answers are provided in Appendix A.

1. The palpebral fissure is:

   a. the border between the cornea and sclera.
   b. the open space between the eyelids.
   c. the angle where the eyelids meet.
   d. visible on the upper and lower lids at the inner canthus.

2. The corneal reflex is mediated by cranial nerves:

   a. II and III.
   b. II and VI.
   c. V and VII.
   d. VI and IV.

3. The retinal structures viewed through the ophthalmoscope are:

   a. the optic disc, the retinal vessels, the general background, and the macula.
   b. the cornea, the lens, the choroid, and the ciliary body.
   c. the optic papilla, the sclera, the retina, and the iris.
   d. the pupil, the sclera, the ciliary body, and the macula.

4. The examiner records "positive consensual light reflex." This is:

   a. the convergence of the axes of the eyeballs.
   b. the simultaneous constriction of the other pupil when one eye is exposed to bright light.
   c. a reflex direction of the eye toward an object attracting a person's attention.
   d. the adaptation of the eye for near vision.

5. Several changes occur in the eye with the aging process. The thickening and yellowing of the lens is referred to as:

   a. presbyopia.
   b. floaters.
   c. macular degeneration.
   d. senile cataract.

6. Be alert to symptoms that may constitute an eye emergency. Identify the symptom(s) that should be referred immediately.

   a. floaters
   b. epiphora
   c. sudden onset of vision change
   d. photophobia

7. Visual acuity is assessed with:

   a. the Snellen eye chart.
   b. an ophthalmoscope.
   c. the Hirschberg test.
   d. the confrontation test.

8. The cover test is used to assess for:

   a. nystagmus.
   b. peripheral vision.
   c. muscle weakness.
   d. visual acuity.

9. When using the ophthalmoscope, you would:

   a. remove your own glasses and approach the patient's left eye with your left eye.
   b. leave light on in the examining room and remove glasses from the patient.
   c. remove glasses and set the diopter setting at 0.
   d. use the smaller white light and instruct the patient to focus on the ophthalmoscope.

10. The six muscles that control eye movement are innervated by cranial nerves:

    a. II, III, V.
    b. IV, VI, VII.
    c. III, IV, VI.
    d. II, III, VI.

11. Conjunctivitis is always associated with:

    a. absent red reflex.
    b. reddened conjunctiva.
    c. impairment of vision.
    d. fever.

12. A patient has blurred peripheral vision. You suspect glaucoma, and test the visual fields. A person with normal vision would see your moving finger temporally at:

    a. 50 degrees.
    b. 60 degrees.
    c. 90 degrees.
    d. 180 degrees.

13. A person is known to be blind in the left eye. What happens to the pupils when the right eye is illuminated by a penlight beam?

    a. No response in both.
    b. Both pupils constrict.
    c. Right pupil constricts, left has no response.
    d. Left pupil constricts, right has no response.

14. Use of the ophthalmoscope: an interruption of the red reflex occurs when:

    a. there is an opacity in the cornea or lens.
    b. the patient has pathology of the optic tract.
    c. the blood vessels are tortuous.
    d. the pupils are constricted.

15. One cause of visual impairment in aging adults is:

    a. strabismus.
    b. glaucoma.
    c. amblyopia.
    d. retinoblastoma.

16. Briefly describe the method of assessing the six cardinal fields of vision.

SKILLS LABORATORY/CLINICAL SETTING

You are now ready for the clinical component of the eye examination. The purpose of the clinical component is to practise the steps of the examination on a peer in the skills laboratory. Note that the first practice session usually takes a long time because there are so many separate steps. Be aware that success with the use of the ophthalmoscope is hard to achieve during the first practice session. Make sure you are holding the instrument correctly and practise focusing on various objects about the room before you try to look at a person's fundus. When you do examine a peer's eye, make sure to offer occasional rest times. It is very tiring for the "patient" to have the ophthalmoscope light shining in the eye. During the first practice session, aim for finding the red reflex and a retinal vessel or two; if you can locate the optic disc, so much the better.

CLINICAL OBJECTIVES

1. Collect a health history related to pertinent signs and symptoms of the eye system.

2. Demonstrate and explain assessment of visual acuity, visual fields, external eye structures, and ocular fundus.

3. Record the history and physical examination findings accurately, reach an assessment of the health state, and develop a plan of care.

INSTRUCTIONS

Prepare the examination setting. Wash your hands. Practise the steps of the examination on a peer in the skills laboratory, giving appropriate instructions as you proceed. Record your findings using the regional write-up sheet that follows. The front of the page is intended as a worksheet; the back of the page is intended for your narrative summary recording using the SOAP format.

REGIONAL WRITE-UP—EYES

Date _____

Examiner _____

Patient _____ Age _____ Gender _____

Occupation _____

I. Health History

	No	Yes, explain
1. Any **difficulty seeing** or blurring?	____	_____
2. Any eye **pain**?	____	_____
3. Any history of **crossed eyes**?	____	_____
4. Any **redness** or **swelling** in eyes?	____	_____
5. Any **watering** or **tearing**?	____	_____
6. Any **injury** or **surgery** to eye?	____	_____
7. Ever tested for **glaucoma**?	____	_____
8. Wear **glasses** or **contact lenses**?	____	_____
9. Ever had vision tested?	____	_____
10. Taking any medications?	____	_____

II. Physical Examination

A. Test visual acuity

Snellen eye chart _____

Pocket vision screener for near vision _____

B. Test visual fields

Confrontation test _____

C. Inspect extraocular muscle function

Corneal light reflex _____

Cover test _____

Diagnostic positions test _____

D. Inspect external eye structures

General _____

Eyebrows _____

Eyelids and lashes _____

Eyeballs _____

Conjunctiva and sclera _____

Lacrimal gland, puncta _____

E. Inspect anterior eyeball structures

Cornea _____

Iris _____

Pupil size _____

Pupil direct and consensual light reflex _____

Accommodation _____

F. Inspect ocular fundus

Optic disc _____

Vessels _____

General background of fundus _____

Macula _____

REGIONAL WRITE-UP—EYES

Summarize your findings using the SOAP format.

Subjective (Reason for seeking care, health history)

Objective (Physical examination findings)

Record findings on diagram below

R

L

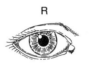 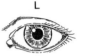

Assessment (Assessment of problem, diagnosis)

Plan (Diagnostic evaluation, follow-up care, teaching)

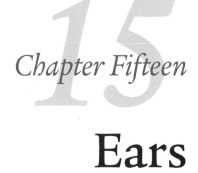

Chapter Fifteen

Ears

PURPOSE

This chapter helps you to learn the structure and function of the ears; to learn the methods of examination of hearing, external ear structures, and tympanic membrane using the otoscope; and to record the assessment accurately.

READING ASSIGNMENT

Jarvis, *Physical Examination and Health Assessment,* 1st Canadian ed., Chapter 15, pp. 341–370.

AUDIO-VISUAL ASSIGNMENT

Jarvis, *Physical Examination and Health Assessment DVD Series: Head, Eyes, and Ears*

GLOSSARY

Study the following terms after completing the reading assignment. You should be able to cover the definition on the right and define the term out loud.

Annulus ....outer fibrous rim encircling the eardrum

Atresia...congenital absence or closure of ear canal

Cerumen......................................yellow waxy material that lubricates and protects the ear canal

Cochlea.......................................inner ear structure containing the central hearing apparatus

Eustachian tube ....connects the middle ear with the nasopharynx and allows passage of air

Helix...superior, posterior free rim of the pinna

Incus ...."anvil," middle of the three ossicles of the middle ear

Malleus ...."hammer," first of the three ossicles of the middle ear

Mastoid.......................................bony prominence of the skull located just behind the ear

Organ of Corti ....sensory organ of hearing

Otalgia ....pain in the ear

Otitis externa ....inflammation of the outer ear and ear canal

Otitis media ....inflammation of the middle ear and tympanic membrane

Otorrhea....................................discharge from the ear

Pars flaccida ....small, slack, superior section of tympanic membrane

Pars tensa ....thick, taut, central/inferior section of tympanic membrane

Pinna ....auricle, or outer ear

Stapes.."stirrup," inner of the three ossicles of the middle ear

Tinnitus....................................ringing in the ears

Tympanic membrane................."eardrum," thin, translucent, oval membrane that stretches across the ear canal and separates the middle ear from the outer ear

Umbo ....knob of the malleus that shows through the tympanic membrane

Vertigo ....a spinning, twirling sensation

STUDY GUIDE

After completing the reading assignment and the audio-visual assignment, you should be able to answer the following questions in the spaces provided.

1. List the three functions of the middle ear.

2. Contrast two pathways of hearing.

3. Differentiate among the types of hearing loss, and give examples.

4. Relate the anatomic differences that place the infant at greater risk for middle ear infections.

5. Describe these tests of hearing acuity: whispered voice test; Weber test; Rinne test.

6. Explain the positioning of normal ear alignment in the child.

7. Define *otosclerosis* and *presbycusis.*

8. Contrast the motions used to straighten the ear canal when using the otoscope with an infant versus an adult.

9. Describe the appearance of these nodules that could be present on the external ear: Darwin's tubercle; sebaceous cyst; tophi; chondrodermatitis; keloid; carcinoma.

10. Describe the appearance of these conditions that could appear in the ear canal: osteoma; exostosis; furuncle; polyp; foreign body.

11. List the disease state suggested by the following descriptions of the appearance of the eardrum:

yellow-amber colour _____

pearly grey colour _____

air-fluid level _____

distorted light reflex _____

red colour _____

dense white areas _____

oval dark areas _____

black or white dots on drum _____

blue drum _____

12. List the findings that may appear during the whispered voice test, the Weber test, and the Rinne test for:

Conductive hearing loss _____.

Sensorineural loss _____.

Fill in the labels indicated on the following illustrations.

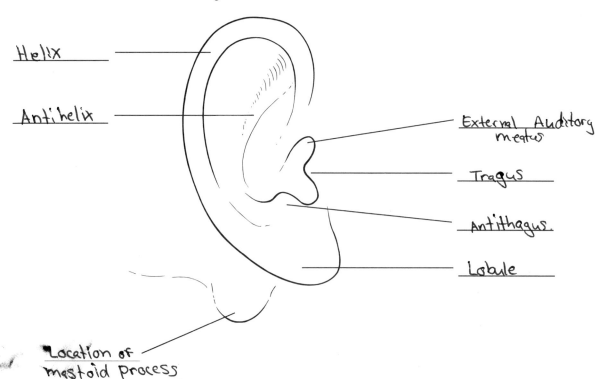

Helix

Antihelix

External Auditory meatus

Tragus

Antithagus

Lobule

Location of mastoid process

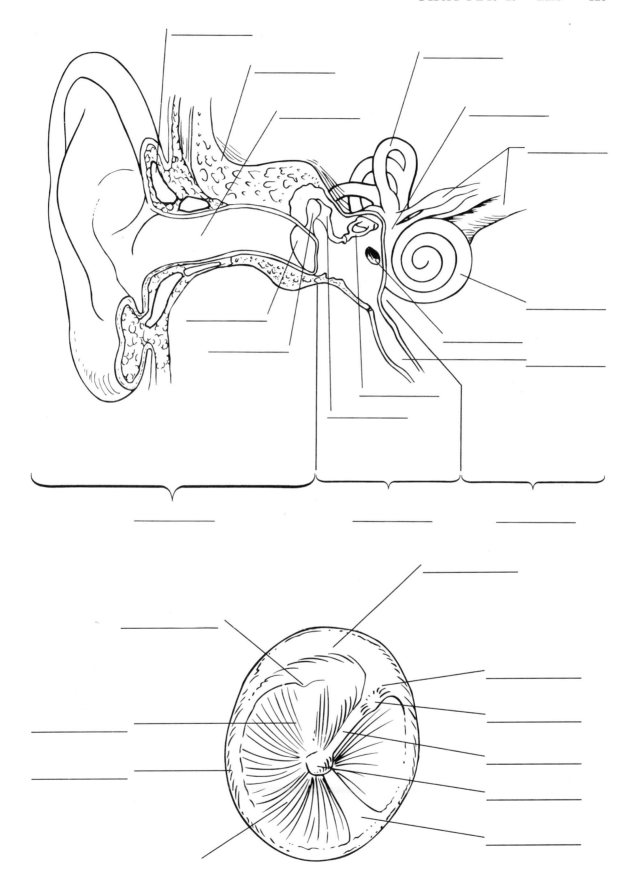

REVIEW QUESTIONS

This test is for you to check your own mastery of the content. Answers are provided in Appendix A.

1. Using the otoscope, the tympanic membrane is visualized. The colour of a normal membrane is:

    a. deep pink.
    b. creamy white.
    c. pearly grey.
    d. dependent upon the ethnicity of the individual.

2. Sensorineural hearing loss may be related to:

    a. a gradual nerve degeneration.
    b. foreign bodies.
    c. impacted cerumen.
    d. perforated tympanic membrane.

3. Prior to examining the ear with the otoscope, the _____ should be palpated for tenderness.

    a. helix, external auditory meatus, and lobule
    b. mastoid process, tympanic membrane, and malleus
    c. pinna, pars flaccida, and antitragus
    d. pinna, tragus, and mastoid process

4. During the otoscopic examination of a child less than three years of age, the examiner:

    a. pulls the pinna up and back.
    b. pulls the pinna down.
    c. holds the pinna gently but firmly in its normal position.
    d. tilts the head slightly toward the examiner.

5. While viewing with the otoscope, the examiner instructs the person to hold the nose and swallow. During this manoeuvre, the eardrum should:

    a. flutter.
    b. retract.
    c. bulge.
    d. remain immobile.

6. To differentiate between air conduction and bone conduction hearing loss, the examiner would perform:

    a. the Weber test.
    b. the Romberg test.
    c. the Rinne test.
    d. the whisper test.

7. In examining the ear of an adult, the canal is straightened by pulling the auricle:

    a. down and forward.
    b. down and back.
    c. up and back.
    d. up and forward.

8. Darwin's tubercle is:

    a. an overgrowth of scar tissue.
    b. a blocked sebaceous gland.
    c. a sign of gout called tophi.
    d. a congenital, painless nodule at the helix.

9. When the ear is being examined with an otoscope, the patient's head should be:

    a. tilted toward the examiner.
    b. titled away from the examiner.
    c. as vertical as possible.
    d. tilted down.

10. The hearing receptors are located in the:

    a. vestibule.
    b. semicircular canals.
    c. middle ear.
    d. cochlea.

11. The sensation of vertigo is the result of:

    a. otitis media.
    b. pathology in the semicircular canals.
    c. pathology in the cochlea.
    d. fourth cranial nerve damage.

12. A common cause of a conductive hearing loss is:

    a. impacted cerumen.
    b. acute rheumatic fever.
    c. a CVA.
    d. otitis externa.

13. In the Rinne test, the 2 to 1 ratio refers to:

    a. the loudness of the tone heard by the two ears.
    b. the lengths of time until the patient stops hearing the tone by air conduction and by bone conduction.
    c. the lengths of time until the patient no longer hears the tone and the examiner no longer hears the tone.
    d. the examiner hearing the tone twice as long as the patient hears it.

14. Upon examination of the tympanic membrane, visualization of which of the following findings indicates acute purulent otitis media infection?

    a. absent light reflex, bluish drum, oval dark areas
    b. absent light reflex, reddened drum, bulging drum
    c. oval dark areas on drum
    d. absent light reflex, air-fluid level, or bubbles behind drum
    e. retracted drum, very prominent landmarks

15. In examining a young adult woman, you observe her tympanic membrane to be yellow in colour. You suspect she has:

    a. serum in the middle ear.
    b. blood in the middle ear.
    c. infection of the drumhead.
    d. jaundice.

16. Risk reduction for acute otitis media includes:

    a. use of pacifiers.
    b. increasing group daycare.
    c. avoiding breastfeeding.
    d. eliminating smoking in the house and car.

SKILLS LABORATORY/CLINICAL SETTING

You are now ready for the clinical component of the ear examination. The purpose of the clinical component is to practise the steps of the ear examination on a peer in the skills laboratory or on a patient in the clinical setting. The use of the otoscope is somewhat easier than the use of the ophthalmoscope; however, you still must be sure you are holding the instrument correctly. Holding the otoscope in an "upside down" position seems awkward at first, but it is important in order to make sure the otoscope tip does not cause pain to the delicate parts of the ear canal. Have someone correct your positioning before you insert the instrument.

CLINICAL OBJECTIVES

1. Collect a health history related to pertinent signs and symptoms of the ear system.

2. Describe the appearance of the normal outer ear and external ear canal.

3. Describe and demonstrate the correct technique of an otoscopic examination.

4. Describe and perform tests for hearing acuity.

5. Systematically describe the normal tympanic membrane including position, colour, and landmarks.

6. Record the history and physical examination findings accurately, reach an assessment about the health state, and develop a plan of care.

INSTRUCTIONS

Prepare the examination setting and gather your equipment. Make certain the otoscope light is bright and batteries are freshly charged. Wash your hands. Practise the steps of the examination on a peer in the skills laboratory, giving appropriate instructions as you proceed. Record your findings using the regional write-up sheet that follows. The front of the page is intended as a worksheet; the back of the page is intended for your narrative summary recording using the SOAP format.

NOTES

REGIONAL WRITE-UP—EARS

Date _____

Examiner _____

Patient _____ Age _____ Gender _____

Occupation _____

I. Health History

	No	Yes, explain
1. Any **earache** or ear pain?	_____	_____
2. Any ear **infections**?	_____	_____
3. Any **discharge** from ears?	_____	_____
4. Any **hearing loss**?	_____	_____
5. Any **loud noises** at home or job?	_____	_____
6. Any **ringing** or **buzzing** in ears?	_____	_____
7. Ever felt **vertigo** (spinning)?	_____	_____
8. How do you clean your ears?	_____	_____

II. Physical Examination

A. Inspect and palpate external ear

Size and shape _____

Skin condition _____

Tenderness _____

External auditory meatus _____

B. Inspect using the otoscope

External canal _____

Tympanic membrane _____

Colour and characteristics _____

Position _____

Integrity of membrane _____

C. Test hearing acuity

Whispered voice test _____

Weber test _____

Rinne test _____

REGIONAL WRITE-UP—EARS

Summarize your findings using the SOAP format.

Subjective (Reason for seeking care, health history)

Objective (Physical examination findings)

Record findings on diagram below

R   L

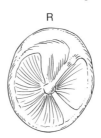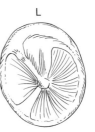

Assessment (Assessment of health state or problem, diagnosis)

Plan (Diagnostic evaluation, follow-up care, patient teaching)

Nose, Mouth, and Throat

PURPOSE

This chapter helps you to learn the structure and function of the nose, mouth, and throat; to learn the methods of inspection and palpation of these structures; and to record the assessment accurately.

READING ASSIGNMENT

Jarvis, *Physical Examination and Health Assessment,* 1st Canadian ed., Chapter 16, pp. 371–404.

AUDIO-VISUAL ASSIGNMENT

Jarvis, *Physical Examination and Health Assessment DVD Series: Nose, Mouth, Throat, and Neck*

GLOSSARY

Study the following terms after completing the reading assignment. You should be able to cover the definition on the right and define the term out loud.

Aphthous ulcers ...."canker sores"—small, painful, round ulcers in the oral mucosa of unknown cause

Buccal ....pertaining to the cheek

Candidiasis ....(moniliasis) white, cheesy, curdlike patch on buccal mucosa due to superficial fungal infection

Caries..decay in the teeth

Crypts ....indentations on surface of tonsils

Cheilitis ....red, scaling, shallow, painful fissures at corners of mouth

Choanal atresia..........................closure of nasal cavity due to congenital septum between nasal cavity and pharynx

Epistaxis ....nosebleed, usually from anterior septum

Epulis................................nontender, fibrous nodule of the gum

Fordyce's granules......................small, isolated, white or yellow papules on oral mucosa

Gingivitis..................................red, swollen gum margins that bleed easily

Herpes simplex............................"cold sores"—clear vesicles with red base that evolve into pustules, usually at lip–skin junction

Koplik's spots.............................small, blue-white spots with red halo over oral mucosa; early sign of measles

Leukoplakia...............................chalky white, thick, raised patch on sides of tongue; precancerous

Malocclusion.............................upper or lower dental arches out of alignment

Papillae..................................rough bumpy elevation on dorsal surface of tongue

Parotid glands............................pair of salivary glands in the cheeks in front of the ears

Pharyngitis................................inflammation of the throat

Plaque...................................soft whitish debris on teeth

Polyp....................................smooth, pale grey nodules in the nasal cavity due to chronic allergic rhinitis

Rhinitis.......................................red swollen inflammation of nasal mucosa

Thrush..oral candidiasis in the newborn

Turbinate...................................one of three bony projections into nasal cavity

Uvula..free projection hanging down from the middle of the soft palate

STUDY GUIDE

After completing the reading assignment and the audio-visual assignment, you should be able to answer the following questions in the spaces provided.

1. Name the functions of the nose.

2. Describe the size and components of the nasal cavity.

3. List the four sets of paranasal sinuses and describe their function.

4. List the three pairs of salivary glands, including their location and the locations of their duct openings.

5. Following tooth loss in the middle-aged or older adult, describe the consequences of chewing with the remaining maloccluded teeth.

6. Describe the appearance of a deviated nasal septum and a perforated septum.

7. Describe the appearance of a torus palatinus and explain its significance.

8. Contrast the physical appearance and clinical significance of: leukoedema; candidiasis; leukoplakia; Fordyce's granules.

9. List the four-point grading scale for the size of tonsils.

10. Describe the appearance and clinical significance of these findings in the infant: sucking tubercle; Epstein's pearls; Bednar aphthae.

11. Contrast the appearance of nasal turbinates versus nasal polyps.

12. Describe the appearance and clinical significance of these findings on the tongue: ankyloglossia; fissured tongue; geographic tongue; black hairy tongue; macroglossia.

13. In the space below, sketch a cleft palate and a bifid uvula.

14. Describe the appearance of oral Kaposi's sarcoma.

Fill in the labels indicated on the following illustrations.

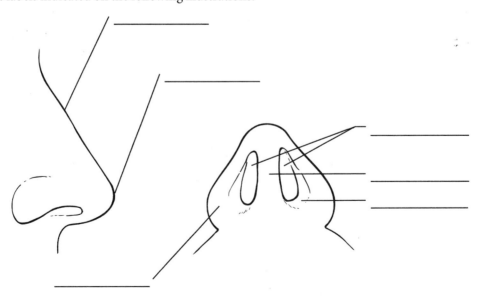

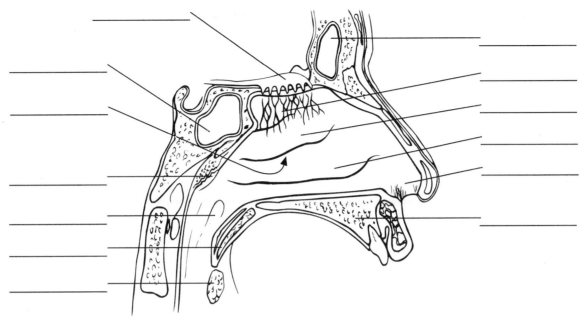

LEFT LATERAL WALL—NASAL CAVITY

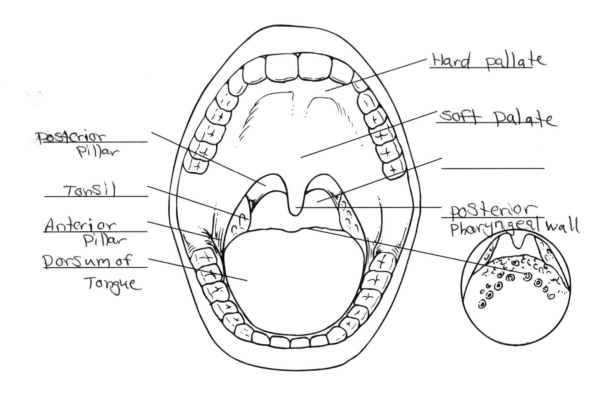

Posterior
Pillar

Tonsil

Anterior
Pillar

Dorsum of
Tongue

Hard pallate

Soft Palate

posterior
Pharyngeal wall

REVIEW QUESTIONS

This test is for you to check your own mastery of the content. Answers are provided in Appendix A.

1. The most common site of nosebleeds is:

    a. the turbinates.
    b. the columellae.
    c. Kiesselbach's plexus.
    d. the meatus.

2. The sinuses that are accessible to examination are the:

    a. ethmoid and sphenoid.
    b. frontal and ethmoid.
    c. maxillary and sphenoid.
    d. frontal and maxillary sinuses.

3. The frenulum is:

    a. the midline fold of tissue that connects the tongue to the floor of the mouth.
    b. the anterior border of the oral cavity.
    c. the arching roof of the mouth.
    d. the free projection hanging down from the middle of the soft palate.

4. The largest salivary gland is located:

    a. within the cheeks in front of the ear.
    b. beneath the mandible at the angle of the jaw.
    c. within the floor of the mouth under the tongue.
    d. at the base of the tongue.

5. A 70-year-old woman complains of dry mouth. The most frequent cause of this problem is:

    a. the aging process.
    b. related to medications she may be taking.
    c. the use of dentures.
    d. related to a diminished sense of smell.

6. Because of a history of headache, the examiner uses transillumination to assess for an inflamed sinus. The findings in a healthy individual would be:

    a. a diffuse red glow.
    b. no transillumination.
    c. findings vary with ethnicity of the person.
    d. light visible in the nares through a speculum.

7. During an inspection of the nares, a deviated septum is noted. The best action is to:

    a. request a consultation with an ear, nose, and throat specialist.
    b. document the deviation in the medical record in case the person needs to be suctioned.
    c. teach the person what to do if a nosebleed should occur.
    d. explore further because polyps frequently accompany a deviated septum.

8. Oral malignancies are most likely to develop:

    a. on the soft palate.
    b. on the tongue.
    c. in the buccal cavity.
    d. under the tongue.

9. In a medical record, the tonsils are graded as 3+. The tonsils would be:

    a. visible.
    b. halfway between the tonsillar pillars and uvula.
    c. touching the uvula.
    d. touching each other.

10. The function of the nasal turbinates is to:

    a. warm the inhaled air.
    b. detect odours.
    c. stimulate tear formation.
    d. lighten the weight of the skull bones.

11. The opening of an adult's parotid gland (Stensen's duct) is opposite the:

    a. lower second molar.
    b. lower incisors.
    c. upper incisors.
    d. upper second molar.

12. A nasal polyp may be distinguished from the nasal turbinates by three of the following characteristics. Which characteristic is *false?*

    a. The polyp is highly vascular.
    b. The polyp is movable.
    c. The polyp is pale grey in colour.
    d. The polyp is nontender.

SKILLS LABORATORY/CLINICAL SETTING

You are now ready for the clinical component of the nose, mouth, and throat examination. The purpose of the clinical component is to practise the steps of the examination on a peer in the skills laboratory or on a patient in the clinical setting and to achieve the following:

CLINICAL OBJECTIVES

1. Inspect the external nose.

2. Demonstrate use of the otoscope and nasal attachment to inspect the structures of the nasal cavity.

3. Demonstrate knowledge of infection control practices during inspection and palpation of structures of the mouth and pharynx.

4. Record the history and physical examination findings accurately, reach an assessment of the health state, and develop a plan of care.

INSTRUCTIONS

Prepare the examination setting and gather your equipment. Wash your hands. Practise the steps of the examination on a peer in the skills laboratory, giving appropriate instructions as you proceed. Record your findings using the regional write-up sheet that follows. The front of the page is intended as a worksheet; the back of the page is intended for your narrative summary recording using the SOAP format.

NOTES

REGIONAL WRITE-UP—NOSE, MOUTH, AND THROAT

Date _____

Examiner _____

Patient _____ Age _____ Gender _____

Occupation _____

I. Health History

	No	Yes, explain
A. Nose		
1. Any nasal **discharge**?		
2. Unusually frequent or severe colds?		
3. Any **sinus pain** or sinusitis?		
4. Any **trauma** or injury to nose?		
5. Any **nosebleeds**? How often?		
6. Any **allergies** or hay fever?		
7. Any change in sense of smell?		
B. Mouth and throat		
1. Any **sores** in mouth, tongue?		
2. Any **sore throat**? How often?		
3. Any **bleeding gums**?		
4. Any **toothache**?		
5. Any **hoarseness,** voice change?		
6. Any difficulty **swallowing**?		
7. Any change in sense of taste?		
8. Do you smoke? How much/day?		
9. Tell me about usual dental care.		

II. Physical Examination

A. Inspect and palpate the nose

Symmetry _____

Deformity, asymmetry, inflammation _____

Test patency of each nostril _____

Using a nasal speculum, note:

    Colour of nasal mucosa _____

    Discharge, foreign body _____

    Septum: deviation, perforation, bleeding _____

    Turbinates: colour, swelling, exudate, polyps _____

B. Palpate the sinus area

Frontal _____

Maxillary _____

C. Inspect the mouth

Lips _____

Teeth and gums _____

Buccal mucosa _____

Palate and uvula _____

Tonsils (grade) _____

Tongue _____

D. Inspect the throat
Tonsils: condition and grade _____

Pharyngeal wall _____

Any breath odour _____

REGIONAL WRITE-UP—NOSE, MOUTH, AND THROAT

Summarize your findings using the SOAP format.

Subjective (Reason for seeking care, health history)

Objective (Physical examination findings)   Record findings on diagram below

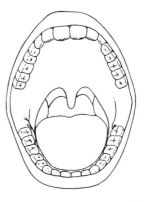

Assessment (Assessment of health state or problem, diagnosis)

Plan (Diagnostic evaluation, follow-up care, patient teaching)

Breasts and Regional Lymphatics

PURPOSE

This chapter helps you to learn the structure and function of the breast, to understand the rationale and methods of examination of the breast, to accurately record the assessment, and to teach breast self-examination.

READING ASSIGNMENT

Jarvis, *Physical Examination and Health Assessment,* 1st Canadian ed., Chapter 17, pp. 405–434.

AUDIO-VISUAL ASSIGNMENT

Jarvis, *Physical Examination and Health Assessment DVD Series: Breasts and Regional Lymphatics*

GLOSSARY

Study the following terms after completing the reading assignment. You should be able to cover the definition on the right and define the term out loud.

Alveoli ....smallest structure of mammary gland

Areola .... darkened area surrounding nipple

Colostrum ....thin, yellow fluid, precursor of milk, secreted for a few days after birth

Cooper's ligaments ....suspensory ligament, fibrous bands extending from the inner breast surface to the chest wall muscles

Fibroadenoma ....benign breast mass

Gynecomastia ....excessive breast development in the male

Intraductal papilloma ....serosanguineous nipple discharge

Inverted ....nipples that are depressed or invaginated

Lactiferous ....conveying milk

Mastitis ....inflammation of the breast

Montgomery's glands ....sebaceous glands in the areola that secrete protective lipid during lactation; also called tubercles of Montgomery

Paget's disease ....intraductal carcinoma in the breast

Peau d'orange ....orange-peel appearance of breast due to edema

Retraction ....dimple or pucker on the skin

Striae ....atrophic pink, purple, or white linear streaks on the breasts, associated with pregnancy, excessive weight gain, or rapid growth during adolescence

Supernumerary nipple ....minute extra nipple along the embryonic milk line

Tail of Spence ....extension of breast tissue into the axilla

STUDY GUIDE

After completing the reading assignment and the audio-visual assignment, you should be able to answer the following questions in the spaces provided.

1. Identify appropriate history questions to ask regarding the breast examination.

2. Describe the anatomy of the breast.

3. Correlate changes in the female breast with normal developmental stages.

4. Describe the components of the breast examination.

5. List points to include in teaching the breast self-examination.

6. Explain the significance of a supernumerary nipple.

7. Differentiate between the female and male breast examination procedure and findings.

8. Discuss pathological changes that may occur in the breast:

   Benign breast disease

   Abscess

   Acute mastitis

   Fibroadenoma

   Cancer

   Paget's disease

9. List and describe the characteristics to consider when a mass is noted in the breast.

10. Define gynecomastia.

11. Describe mammography and clinical breast examination for diagnosis of breast lesions.

12. List the high-risk and moderate-risk factors that increase the usual risk of breast cancer.

Fill in the labels on the following diagrams.

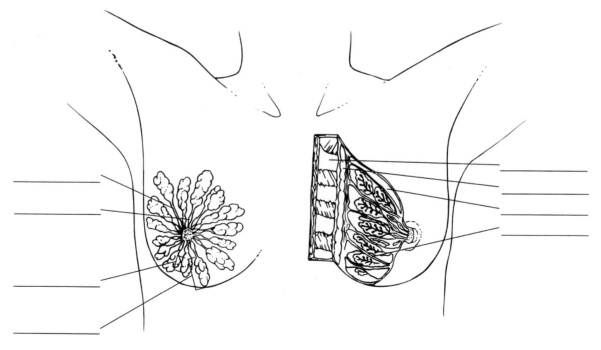

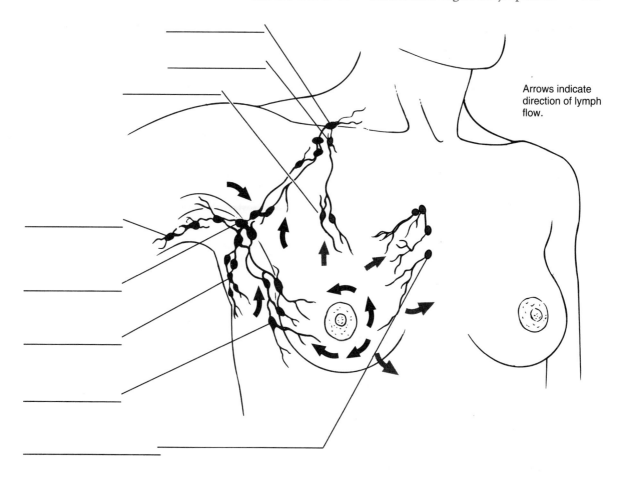

Arrows indicate direction of lymph flow.

REVIEW QUESTIONS

This test is for you to check your own mastery of the content. Answers are provided in Appendix A.

1. The reservoirs for storing milk in the breast are:

   a. lobules.
   b. alveoli.
   c. Montgomery's glands.
   d. lactiferous sinuses.

2. The most common site of breast tumours is:

   a. upper inner quadrant.
   b. upper outer quadrant.
   c. lower inner quadrant.
   d. lower outer quadrant.

3. During a visit for a school physical, the 13-year-old girl being examined questions the asymmetry of her breasts. The best response is:

   a. "One breast may grow faster than the other during development."
   b. "I will give you a referral for a mammogram."
   c. "You will probably have fibrocystic disease when you are older."
   d. "This may be an indication of hormonal imbalance. We will check again in six months."

4. When teaching the breast self-examination, you would inform the woman that the best time to conduct breast self-examination is:

   a. at the onset of the menstrual period.
   b. on the 14th day of the menstrual cycle.
   c. on the 4th to 7th day of the cycle.
   d. just before the menstrual period.

5. In Canada, a screening mammogram is recommended:

   a. every year for women age 40 to 65 years.
   b. every two years for women age 50 to 69 years.
   c. twice a year for all women.
   d. only the baseline examination is needed unless the woman has symptoms.

6. The examiner is going to inspect the breasts for retraction. The best position for this part of the examination is:

   a. lying supine with arms at the sides.
   b. leaning forward with hands outstretched.
   c. sitting with hands pushing onto hips.
   d. one arm at the side, the other arm elevated.

7. A bimanual technique may be the preferred approach for a woman:

   a. who is pregnant.
   b. who is having the first breast examination by a healthcare provider.
   c. with pendulous breasts.
   d. who has felt a change in the breast during self-examination.

8. During the examination of a 70-year-old man, you note gynecomastia. You would:

   a. refer for a biopsy.
   b. refer for a mammogram.
   c. review the medications for drugs that have gynecomastia as a side effect.
   d. proceed with the examination. This is a normal part of the aging process.

9. During a breast examination, you detect a mass. Identify the description that is most consistent with cancer rather than benign breast disease.

   a. round, firm, well demarcated
   b. irregular, poorly defined, fixed
   c. rubbery, mobile, tender
   d. lobular, clear margins, negative skin retraction

10. During the examination of the breasts of a pregnant woman, you would expect to find:

    a. peau d'orange.
    b. nipple retraction.
    c. a unilateral, obvious venous pattern.
    d. a blue vascular pattern over both breasts.

11. Which of the following women should not be referred to a physician for further evaluation?

    a. a 26-year-old with multiple nodules palpated in each breast
    b. a 48-year-old who has a six-month history of reddened and sore left nipple and areolar area
    c. a 25-year-old with asymmetrical breasts and inversion of nipples since adolescence
    d. a 64-year-old with ulcerated area at tip of right nipple, no masses, tenderness, or lymph nodes palpated

12. Breast asymmetry:

    a. increases with age and parity.
    b. may be normal.
    c. indicates a neoplasm.
    d. is accompanied by enlarged axillary lymph nodes.

13. Any lump found in the breast should be referred for further evaluation. A benign lesion will usually have three of the following characteristics. Which one is characteristic of a malignant lesion?

    a. soft
    b. well-defined margins
    c. freely movable
    d. irregular shape

14. Gynecomastia is:

    a. enlargement of the male breast.
    b. presence of "mast" cells in the male breast.
    c. cancer of the male breast.
    d. presence of supernumerary breast on the male chest.

15. Which is the first physical change associated with puberty in girls?

    a. areolar elevation
    b. breast bud development
    c. height spurt
    d. pubic hair development
    e. menarche

SKILLS LABORATORY/CLINICAL SETTING

You are now ready for the clinical component of the breast assessment. The purpose of the clinical component is to practise the steps of the assessment on a peer in the skills laboratory and to achieve the following:

CLINICAL OBJECTIVES

1. Demonstrate knowledge of the symptoms related to the breasts and axillae by obtaining a health history.

2. Perform inspection and palpation of the breasts, with the woman in sitting and supine positions, using proper technique and providing appropriate draping.

3. Teach the breast self-examination to a woman or list the points to include in teaching the breast self-examination.

4. Record the history and physical examination findings accurately, reach an assessment of the health state, and develop a plan of care.

INSTRUCTIONS

Practise the steps of the breast examination on a peer or on a woman in the clinical area. Record your findings on the regional write-up sheet that follows. The front of the page is intended as a worksheet; the back of the page is intended for your narrative summary recording using the SOAP format.

Note the student performance checklist that follows the regional write-up sheet. It lists the essential behaviours you should display as an examiner, and it may be used by your clinical instructor to evaluate your clinical teaching of breast self-examination.

NOTES

REGIONAL WRITE-UP—BREASTS AND AXILLAE

Date _____

Examiner _____

Patient _____ Age _____ Gender _____

Occupation _____

I. Health History

	No	Yes, explain
1. Any **pain** or tenderness in breasts?		
2. Any **lump** or thickening in breasts?		
3. Any **discharge** from nipples?		
4. Any **rash** on breasts?		
5. Any **swelling** in the breasts?		
6. Any **trauma** or injury to breasts?		
7. Any **history** of breast disease?		
8. Ever had **surgery** on breasts?		
9. Ever been taught breast self-examination?		
10. Ever had mammography?		

II. Physical Examination

A. Inspection

1. Breasts

Symmetry _____

Skin colour and condition _____

Texture _____

Lesions _____

2. Areolae and nipples

Shape _____

Direction _____

Surface characteristics _____

Discharge _____

3. Response to arm movement _____

4. Axillae _____

B. Palpation

1. Breasts

Texture _____

Masses _____

Tenderness _____

2. Areolae and nipples

Masses _____

Discharge _____

3. Axillae and lymph nodes

Size _____

Shape _____

Consistency _____

Mobility _____

Discrete or matted _____

Tenderness _____

C. Discuss risks and benefits of breast self-examination (BSE) and teach BSE if requested.

REGIONAL WRITE-UP—BREASTS AND AXILLAE

Summarize your findings using the SOAP format.

Subjective (Reason for seeking care, health history)

Objective (Physical examination findings)   Record findings on diagram below

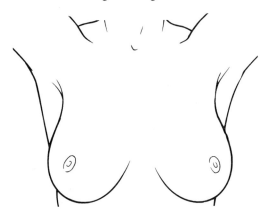

Assessment (Assessment of health state or problem, diagnosis)

Plan (Diagnostic evaluation, follow-up care, teaching)

STUDENT COMPETENCY CHECKLIST

TEACHING BREAST SELF-EXAMINATION (BSE)

	S	U	Comments

A. Cognitive
  1. Explain:
    a. why breasts are examined			

(1) in the shower			
(2) before a mirror			
(3) supine with pillow under side of breast being examined			
b. who should do breast examination			
c. frequency of breast examination			
d. best time of the month to do breast examination and rationale			
2. State the area of breast where most lumps are found			
3. Give two reasons a person may not report significant findings to the healthcare provider			
B. Performance			
1. Explains to woman risks and benefits of BSE			

2. Instructs woman on technique of BSE by:
     a. inspecting and bilaterally comparing breasts in
        front of mirror			

b. noting new or unusual rash or redness on skin and areola			
c. palpating breast in a systemic manner, using pads of three fingers and with woman's arm raised overhead			
d. palpating tail of Spence and axilla			
e. gently compressing nipples			
3. Instructs woman to report unusual findings to the health professional at once			
4. Asks woman to do return demonstration			

NOTES

Chapter Eighteen

Thorax and Lungs

PURPOSE

This chapter helps you to learn the structure and function of the thorax and lungs, to understand the methods of examination of the respiratory system, to identify lung sounds that are normal, to describe the characteristics of adventitious lung sounds, and to accurately record the assessment. At the end of this unit you will be able to perform a complete physical examination of the respiratory system.

READING ASSIGNMENT

Jarvis, *Physical Examination and Health Assessment*, 1st Canadian ed., Chapter 18, pp. 435–478.

AUDIO-VISUAL ASSIGNMENT

Jarvis, *Physical Examination and Health Assessment DVD Series: Thorax and Lungs*

GLOSSARY

Study the following terms after completing the reading assignment. You should be able to cover the definition on the right and define the term out loud.

Alveoli..functional units of the lung; the thin-walled chambers surrounded by networks of capillaries that are the site of respiratory exchange of carbon dioxide and oxygen

Angle of Louis............................manubriosternal angle, the articulation of the manubrium and body of the sternum, continuous with the second rib

Apnea..cessation of breathing

Asthma.......................................an abnormal respiratory condition associated with allergic hypersensitivity to certain inhaled allergens, characterized by bronchospasm, wheezing, and dyspnea

Atelectasis..................................an abnormal respiratory condition characterized by collapsed, shrunken, deflated section of alveoli

Bradypnea..................................slow breathing, <10 breaths per minute, regular rate

Bronchiole ....one of the smaller respiratory passageways into which the segmental bronchi divide

Bronchitis ....inflammation of the bronchi with partial obstruction of bronchi due to excessive mucus secretion

Bronchophony...........................the spoken voice sound heard through the stethoscope, which sounds soft, muffled, and indistinct over normal lung tissue

Bronchovesicular ....the normal breath sound heard over major bronchi, characterized by moderate pitch and an equal duration of inspiration and expiration

Chronic obstructive pulmonary disease (COPD) ......a functional category of abnormal respiratory conditions characterized by airflow obstruction; for example, emphysema and chronic bronchitis

Cilia...millions of hairlike cells lining the tracheobronchial tree

Consolidation............................the solidification of portions of lung tissue as it fills up with infectious exudate, as in pneumonia

Crackles.....................................(rales) abnormal, discontinuous, adventitious lung sounds heard on inspiration

Crepitus.....................................coarse, crackling sensation palpable over the skin when air abnormally escapes from the lung and enters the subcutaneous tissue

Dead space.................................passageways that transport air but are not available for gaseous exchange; for example, trachea and bronchi

Dyspnea.....................................difficult, laboured breathing

Egophony ....the voice sound of "eeeeee" heard through the stethoscope

Emphysema................................the chronic obstructive pulmonary disease characterized by enlargement of alveoli distal to terminal bronchioles

Fissure ....the narrow crack dividing the lobes of the lungs

Fremitus ....a palpable vibration from the spoken voice felt over the chest wall

Friction rub...............................a coarse, grating, adventitious lung sound heard when the pleurae are inflamed

Hypercapnia ....(hypercarbia) increased levels of carbon dioxide in the blood

Hyperventilation.......................increased rate and depth of breathing

Hypoxemia................................decreased level of oxygen in the blood

Intercostal space........................space between the ribs

Kussmaul's respiration..............a type of hyperventilation that occurs with diabetic ketoacidosis

Orthopnea.................................ability to breathe easily only in an upright position

Paroxysmal nocturnal dyspnea ....sudden awakening from sleeping with shortness of breath

Percussion..................................striking over the chest wall with short sharp blows of the fingers in order to determine the size and density of the underlying organ

Pleural effusion ....abnormal fluid between the layers of the pleura

Rhonchi ....low-pitched, musical, snoring, adventitious lung sound caused by airflow obstruction from secretions

Tachypnea ....rapid, shallow breathing, >24 breaths per minute

Vesicular ....the soft, low-pitched, normal breath sounds heard over peripheral lung fields

Vital capacity ....the amount of air, following maximal inspiration, that can be exhaled

Wheeze ....high-pitched, musical, squeaking, adventitious lung sound

Whispered pectoriloquy............a whispered phrase heard through the stethoscope that sounds faint and inaudible over normal lung tissue

Xiphoid process.........................sword-shaped lower tip of the sternum

Study Guide

After completing the reading assignment and the audio-visual assignment, you should be able to answer the following questions in the spaces provided.

1. Describe the most important points about the health history for the respiratory system.

2. Describe the pleura and its function.

3. List the structures that compose the respiratory dead space.

4. Summarize the mechanics of respiration.

5. List the elements included in the inspection of the respiratory system.

6. Discuss the significance of a "barrel chest."

7. List and describe common thoracic deformities.

8. List and describe three types of normal breath sounds.

9. Define two types of adventitious breath sounds.

10. The manubriosternal angle is also called _____.

    Why is it a useful landmark?

11. How many degrees is the normal costal angle? _____.

12. When comparing the anteroposterior diameter of the chest to the transverse diameter, what is the expected ratio?

    What is the significance of this?

13. What is the tripod position?

14. List three factors that affect the normal intensity of tactile fremitus.

    1.

    2.

    3.

15. During percussion, which sound would you expect to predominate over normal lung tissue?

16. Normal findings for diaphragmatic excursion are:

17. List five factors that can cause extraneous noise during auscultation.

    1.

    2.

    3.

    4.

    5.

18. Describe the three types of normal breath sounds:

Name   Location   Description

_____

_____

_____

Fill in the labels indicated on the following illustrations.

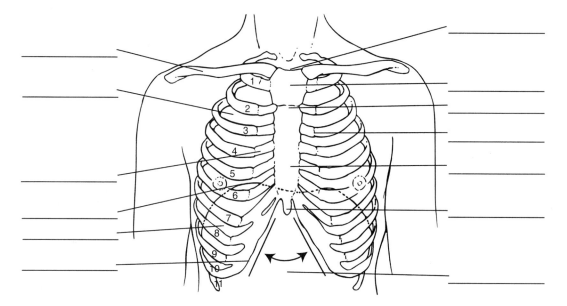

Draw in the lobes of the lungs and label their landmarks on the following two illustrations.

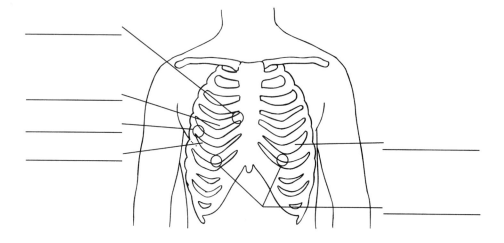

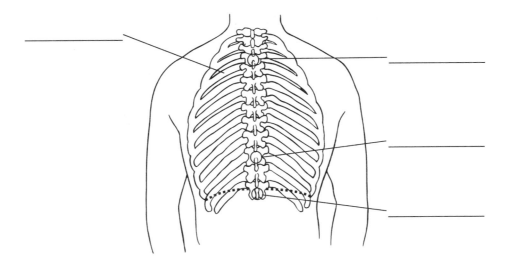

REVIEW QUESTIONS

This test is for you to check your own mastery of the content. Answers are provided in Appendix A.

1. The manubriosternal angle is:

   a. the articulation of the manubrium and the body of the sternum.
   b. a hollow, U-shaped depression just above the sternum.
   c. also known as the breastbone.
   d. a term synonymous with costochondral junction.

2. Select the correct description of the left lung.

   a. narrower than the right lung with three lobes
   b. narrower than the right with two lobes
   c. wider than the right lung with two lobes
   d. shorter than the right with three lobes

3. Some conditions have a cough with characteristic timing. The cough associated with chronic bronchitis is best described as:

   a. continuous throughout the day.
   b. productive cough for at least three months of the year for two years in a row.
   c. occurring in the afternoon or evening because of exposure to irritants at work.
   d. occurring in the early morning.

4. Symmetric chest expansion is best confirmed by:

   a. placing hands on the posterolateral chest wall with thumbs at the level of T9 or T10, then sliding the hands up to pinch a small fold of skin between the thumbs.
   b. inspection of the shape and configuration of the chest wall.
   c. placing the palmar surface of the fingers of one hand against the chest and having the person repeat the words "ninety-nine."
   d. percussion of the posterior chest.

5. Absence of diaphragmatic excursion occurs with:

   a. asthma.
   b. an unusually thick chest wall.
   c. pleural effusion or atelectasis of the lower lobes.
   d. age-related changes in the chest wall.

6. Auscultation of breath sounds is an important component of respiratory assessment. Select the most accurate description of this part of the examination.

   a. Hold the bell of the stethoscope against the chest wall, listen to the entire right field, then the entire left field.
   b. Hold the diaphragm of the stethoscope against the chest wall; listen to one full respiration in each location, being sure to do side-to-side comparisons.
   c. Listen from the apices to the bases of each lung field using the bell of the stethoscope.
   d. Select the bell or diaphragm depending upon the quality of sounds heard; listen for one respiration in each location, moving from side to side.

7. Select the best description of bronchovesicular breath sounds:

   a. high-pitched, of longer duration on inspiration than expiration.
   b. moderate pitch, inspiration equal to expiration.
   c. low-pitched, inspiration greater than expiration.
   d. rustling sound, like the wind in the trees.

8. After examining a patient, you make the following notation: Increased respiratory rate, chest expansion decreased on left side, dull to percussion over left lower lobe, breath sounds louder with fine crackles over left lower lobe. These findings are consistent with a diagnosis of:

   a. bronchitis.
   b. asthma.
   c. pleural effusion.
   d. lobar pneumonia.

9. Upon examining a patient's nails, you note that the angle of the nail base is >160 degrees and that the nail base feels spongy to palpation. These findings are consistent with:

   a. adult respiratory distress syndrome.
   b. normal findings for the nails.
   c. chronic, congenital heart disease and COPD.
   d. atelectasis.

10. Upon examination of a patient, you note a coarse, low-pitched sound during both inspiration and expiration. This patient complains of pain with breathing. These findings are consistent with:

    a. fine crackles.
    b. wheezes.
    c. atelectatic crackles.
    d. pleural friction rub.

11. In order to use the technique of egophony, ask the patient to:

    a. take several deep breaths, then hold for five seconds.
    b. say "eeeeee" each time the stethoscope is moved.
    c. repeat the phrase "ninety-nine" each time the stethoscope is moved.
    d. whisper a phrase as auscultation is performed.

12. When examining for tactile fremitus, it is important to:

    a. have the patient breathe quickly.
    b. ask the patient to cough.
    c. palpate the chest symmetrically.
    d. use the bell of the stethoscope.

13. The pulse oximeter measures:

    a. arterial oxygen saturation.
    b. venous oxygen saturation.
    c. combined saturation of arterial and venous blood.
    d. carboxyhemoglobin levels.

Match column A to column B.

Column A—Lung Borders	Column B—Location
14. _____ apex	a. rests on the diaphragm
15. _____ base	b. C7
16. _____ lateral left	c. sixth rib, midclavicular line
17. _____ lateral right	d. fifth intercostal
18. _____ posterior apex	e. 3 to 4 cm above the inner third of the clavicles

Match column A to column B.

Column A—Configurations of the Thorax	Column B—Description
19. _____ normal chest	a. anteroposterior five transverse diameter
20. _____ barrel chest	b. exaggerated posterior curvature of thoracic spine
21. _____ pectus excavatum	c. lateral, S-shaped curvature of the thoracic and lumbar spine
22. _____ pectus carinatum	d. sunken sternum and adjacent cartilages
23. _____ scoliosis	e. elliptical shape with an anteroposterior to transverse diameter in the ratio of 1:2
24. _____ kyphosis	f. forward protrusion of the sternum with ribs sloping back at either side

SKILLS LABORATORY/CLINICAL SETTING

You are now ready for the clinical component of the respiratory system. The purpose of the clinical component is to practise the regional examination on a peer in the skills laboratory or on a patient in the clinical setting and to achieve the following:

CLINICAL OBJECTIVES

1. Demonstrate knowledge of the symptoms related to the respiratory system by obtaining a regional health history from a peer or patient.

2. Correctly locate anatomic landmarks on the thorax of a peer.

3. Using a grease pencil, and with peer's permission, draw lobes of the lungs on a peer's thorax.

4. Demonstrate correct techniques for inspection, palpation, percussion, and auscultation of the respiratory system.

5. Demonstrate the technique for estimation of diaphragmatic excursion.

6. Record the history and physical examination findings accurately, reach an assessment of the health state, and develop a plan of care.

INSTRUCTIONS

Gather your equipment. Wash your hands. Clean the stethoscope endpiece with an alcohol wipe. Practise the steps of the examination of the thorax and lungs on a peer or on a patient in the clinical area. Record your findings using the regional write-up sheet. The front of the sheet is intended as a worksheet; the back of the sheet is intended for a narrative summary using the SOAP format.

NOTES

REGIONAL WRITE-UP—THORAX AND LUNGS

Date _____

Examiner _____

Patient _____ Age _____ Gender _____

Occupation _____

I. Health History

	No	Yes, explain
1. Do you have a **cough?**		
2. Any shortness of **breath?**		
3. Any **chest pain** with breathing?		
4. Any **past history** of lung diseases?		
5. **Smoke** cigarettes? How many/day?		
6. Any living or work conditions that affect your breathing?		
7. Last TB skin test, chest X-ray, flu vaccine?		

II. Physical Examination

A. Inspection
1. Thoracic cage _____
2. Respiratory rate and pattern _____
3. Skin _____
4. Person's position _____
5. Person's facial expression _____
6. Level of consciousness _____

B. Palpation
1. Confirm symmetrical chest expansion _____
2. Tactile fremitus _____
3. Detect any lumps, masses, tenderness _____
4. Trachea _____

C. Percussion
1. Determine percussion note that predominates over lung fields _____
2. Diaphragmatic excursion _____

D. Auscultation
1. Listen: posterior, lateral, anterior _____
2. Any abnormal breath sounds? _____
   If so, perform bronchophony, _____
   whispered pectoriloquy, _____
   egophony _____
3. Any adventitious sounds? _____

REGIONAL WRITE-UP—THORAX AND LUNGS

Summarize your findings using the SOAP format.

Subjective (Reason for seeking care, health history)

Objective (Physical examination findings)   Use the drawing to record your findings

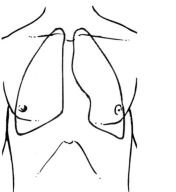 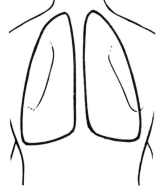

Assessment (Assessment of health state or problem, diagnosis)

Plan (Diagnostic evaluation, follow-up care, teaching)

Heart and Neck Vessels

PURPOSE

This chapter helps you to learn the structure and function of the heart, valves, and great vessels; to understand the cardiac cycle; to describe the heart sounds; to understand the rationale and methods of examination of the heart; and to accurately record the assessment. At the end of this chapter you should be able to perform a complete assessment of the heart and neck vessels.

READING ASSIGNMENT

Jarvis, *Physical Examination and Health Assessment,* 1st Canadian ed., Chapter 19, pp. 479–525.

_____

AUDIO-VISUAL ASSIGNMENT

Jarvis, *Physical Examination and Health Assessment DVD Series: Cardiovascular System: Heart and Neck Vessels*
Google the term *heart sounds.* Listen to several web sites for a good sampling of the most common heart sounds you will encounter.

_____

GLOSSARY

Study the following terms after completing the reading assignment. You should be able to cover the definition on the right and define the term out loud.

Angina pectoris ....acute chest pain that occurs when myocardial demand exceeds its oxygen supply

Aortic regurgitation..................(aortic insufficiency) incompetent aortic valve that allows backward flow of blood into left ventricle during diastole

Aortic stenosis ....calcification of aortic valve cusps that restricts forward flow of blood during systole

Aortic valve ....the left semilunar valve separating the left ventricle and the aorta

Apex of the heart ....tip of the heart pointing down toward the fifth left intercostal space

Apical impulse ....(point of maximal impulse, PMI) pulsation created as the left ventricle rotates against the chest wall during systole, normally at the fifth left intercostal space in the midclavicular line

Base of the heart ....broader area of heart's outline located at the third right and left intercostal space

Bell (of the stethoscope) ....cup-shaped endpiece used for soft, low-pitched heart sounds

Bradycardia ....slow heart rate, <50 beats per minute in the adult

Clubbing.....................................bulbous enlargement of distal phalanges of fingers and toes that occurs with chronic cyanotic heart and lung conditions

Coarctation of aorta...................severe narrowing of the descending aorta, a congenital heart defect

Cor pulmonale...........................right ventricular hypertrophy and heart failure due to pulmonary hypertension

Cyanosis ....dusky blue mottling of the skin and mucous membranes due to excessive amount of reduced hemoglobin in the blood

Diaphragm (of the stethoscope) ....flat endpiece of the stethoscope used for hearing relatively high-pitched heart sounds

Diastole ....the heart's filling phase

Dyspnea.....................................difficult, laboured breathing

Edema ....swelling of legs or dependent body part due to increased interstitial fluid

Erb's point ....traditional auscultatory area in the third left intercostal space

First heart sound (S_1).................occurs with closure of the atrioventricular (AV) valves, signalling the beginning of systole

Fourth heart sound (S_4).............(S_4 gallop; atrial gallop) very soft, low-pitched, ventricular filling sound that occurs in late diastole

Gallop rhythm ....the addition of a third or a fourth heart sound makes the rhythm sound like the cadence of a galloping horse

Inching ....technique of moving the stethoscope incrementally across the precordium through the auscultatory areas while listening to the heart sounds

LVH (left ventricular hypertrophy) ....increase in thickness of myocardial wall that occurs when the heart pumps against chronic outflow obstruction; for example, aortic stenosis

MCL (midclavicular line) ....imaginary vertical line bisecting the middle of the clavicle in each hemithorax

Mitral regurgitation ....(mitral insufficiency) incompetent mitral valve allows regurgitation of blood back into left atrium during systole

Mitral stenosis ....calcified mitral valve impedes forward flow of blood into left ventricle during diastole

Mitral valve ....left AV valve separating the left atria and ventricle

Palpitation ....uncomfortable awareness of rapid or irregular heart rate

Paradoxical splitting.................opposite of a normal split S_2 so that the split is heard in expiration, and in inspiration the sounds fuse to one sound

Pericardial friction rub ....high-pitched scratchy extracardiac sound heard when the precordium is inflamed

Physiological splitting...............normal variation in S_2 heard as two separate components during inspiration

Precordium ....area of the chest wall overlying the heart and great vessels

Pulmonic regurgitation ....(pulmonic insufficiency) backflow of blood through incompetent pulmonic valve into the right ventricle

Pulmonic stenosis ....calcification of pulmonic valve that restricts forward flow of blood during systole

Pulmonic valve ....right semilunar valve separating the right ventricle and pulmonary artery

Second heart sound (S_2) ....occurs with closure of the semilunar valves, aortic and pulmonic, and signals the end of systole

Summation gallop......................abnormal mid-diastolic heart sound heard when both the pathological S_3 and S_4 are present

Syncope.......................................(fainting) temporary loss of consciousness due to decreased cerebral blood flow, caused by ventricular asystole, pronounced bradycardia, or ventricular fibrillation

Systole..the heart's pumping phase

Tachycardia ....rapid heart rate, >100 beats per minute in the adult

Third heart sound (S_3) ....soft, low-pitched, ventricular filling sound that occurs in early diastole (S_3 gallop) and may be an early sign of heart failure

Thrill...palpable vibration on the chest wall accompanying severe heart murmur

Tricuspid valve...........................right AV valve separating the right atria and ventricle

STUDY GUIDE

After completing the reading assignment and the audio-visual assignment, you should be able to answer the following questions in the spaces provided.

1. Define the apical impulse and describe its normal location, size, and duration.

Which *normal* variations may affect the location of the apical impulse?

Which *abnormal* conditions may affect the location of the apical impulse?

2. Explain the mechanism producing normal first and second heart sounds.

3. Describe the effect of respiration on the heart sounds.

4. Describe the characteristics of the first heart sound and its intensity at the apex of the heart and at the base.

Which conditions *increase* the intensity of S_1?

Which conditions *decrease* the intensity of S_1?

5. Describe the characteristics of the second heart sound and its intensity at the apex of the heart and at the base.

Which conditions *increase* the intensity of S_2?

Which conditions *decrease* the intensity of S_2?

6. Explain the physiological mechanism for normal splitting of S_2 in the pulmonic valve area.

7. Define the third heart sound. When in the cardiac cycle does it occur? Describe its intensity, quality, location in which it is heard, and method of auscultation.

8. Differentiate a physiological S_3 from a pathological S_3.

9. Define the fourth heart sound. When in the cardiac cycle does it occur? Describe its intensity, quality, location in which it is heard, and method of auscultation.

10. Explain the position of the valves during each phase of the cardiac cycle.

11. Define venous pressure and jugular venous pulse.

12. Differentiate between the carotid artery pulsation and the jugular vein pulsation.

13. List the areas of questioning to address during the health history for the cardiovascular system.

14. Define bruit, and discuss what it indicates.

15. Define heave or lift, and discuss what it indicates.

16. State four guidelines to distinguish S_1 from S_2.

   1. _____

   2. _____

   3. _____

   4. _____

17. Define pulse deficit, and discuss what it indicates.

18. Define preload and afterload.

19. List the characteristics to explore when you hear a murmur, including the grading scale of murmurs.

20. Discuss the characteristics of an innocent or functional murmur.

Fill in the labels indicated on the following illustrations.

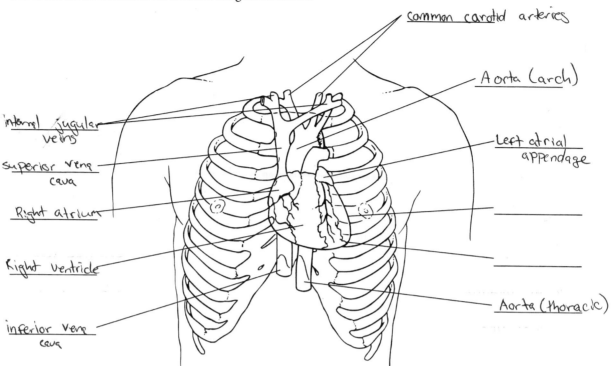

common carotid arteries

Aorta (arch)

internal jugular veins

superior vena cava

Right atrium

Right Ventricle

inferior vena cava

Left atrial appendage

Aorta (thoracic)

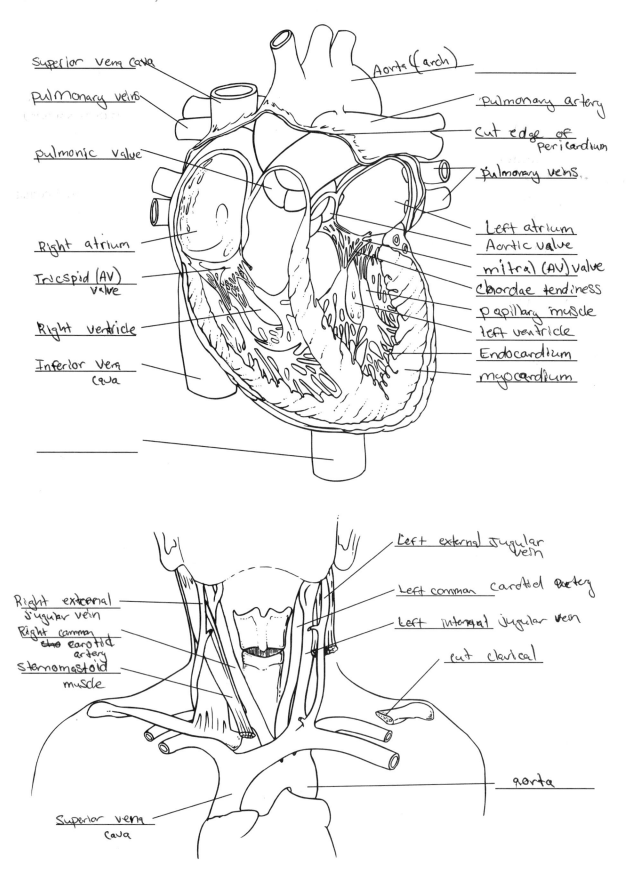

Superior vena cava

Pulmonary veins

pulmonic valve

Right atrium

Tricspid (AV) valve

Right ventricle

Inferior Vena cava

Aorta (arch)

Pulmonary artery

Cut edge of pericardium

Pulmonary veins.

Left atrium

Aortic valve

mitral (AV) valve

Chordae tendiness

Papillary muscle

left ventricle

Endocardium

myocardium

Right external jugular vein

Right comman the carotid artery

Sternomastoid muscle

Left external jugular vein

Left comman carotid artery

Left internal jugular vein

cut clavical

aorta

Superior vena cava

REVIEW QUESTIONS

This test is for you to check your own mastery of the content. Answers are provided in Appendix A.

1. The precordium is:

   a. a synonym for the mediastinum.
   b. the area on the chest where the apical impulse is felt.
   c. the area on the anterior chest overlying the heart and great vessels.
   d. a synonym for the area where the superior and inferior venae cavae return unoxygenated venous blood to the right side of the heart.

2. Select the best description of the tricuspid valve.

   a. left semilunar valve
   b. right atrioventricular valve
   c. left atrioventricular valve
   d. right semilunar valve

3. The function of the pulmonic valve is to:

   a. divide the left atrium and left ventricle.
   b. guard the opening between the right atrium and right ventricle.
   c. protect the orifice between the right ventricle and the pulmonary artery.
   d. guard the entrance to the aorta from the left ventricle.

4. Atrial systole occurs:

   a. during ventricular systole.
   b. during ventricular diastole.
   c. concurrently with ventricular systole.
   d. independently of ventricular function.

5. The second heart sound is the result of:

   a. opening of the mitral and tricuspid valves.
   b. closing of the mitral and tricuspid valves.
   c. opening of the aortic and pulmonic valves.
   d. closing of the aortic and pulmonic valves.

6. The examiner has estimated the jugular venous pressure. Identify the finding that is abnormal.

   a. Patient elevated to 30 degrees, internal jugular vein pulsation at 1 cm above sternal angle
   b. Patient elevated to 30 degrees, internal jugular vein pulsation at 2 cm above sternal angle
   c. Patient elevated to 40 degrees, internal jugular vein pulsation at 1 cm above sternal angle
   d. Patient elevated to 45 degrees, internal jugular vein pulsation at 4 cm above sternal angle

7. The examiner is palpating the apical impulse. The normal size of this impulse:

   a. is less than 1 cm.
   b. is about 2 cm.
   c. is 3 cm.
   d. varies depending on the size of the person.

8. The examiner wishes to listen in the pulmonic valve area. To do this, the stethoscope would be placed at the:

   a. second right interspace.
   b. second left interspace.
   c. left lower sternal border.
   d. fifth interspace, left midclavicular line.

9. Select the statement that best differentiates a split S_2 from S_3.

   a. S_3 is lower pitched and is heard at the apex.
   b. S_2 is heard at the left lower sternal border.
   c. The timing of S_2 varies with respirations.
   d. S_3 is heard at the base; timing varies with respirations.

10. The examiner wishes to listen for a pericardial friction rub. Select the best method of listening.

    a. with the diaphragm, patient sitting up and leaning forward, breath held in expiration
    b. using the bell with the patient leaning forward
    c. at the base during normal respiration
    d. with the diaphragm, patient turned to the left side

11. When auscultating the heart, your first step is to:

    a. identify S_1 and S_2.
    b. listen for S_3 and S_4.
    c. listen for murmurs.
    d. identify all four sounds on the first round.

12. You will hear a split S_2 most clearly in what area?

    a. apical
    b. pulmonic
    c. tricuspid

    d. aortic

13. The stethoscope bell should be pressed lightly against the skin so that:

    a. chest hair does not simulate crackles.
    b. high-pitched sounds can be heard better.
    c. it does not act as a diaphragm.
    d. it does not interfere with amplification of heart sounds.

14. A murmur heard after S_1 and before S_2 is classified as:

    a. diastolic (possibly benign).
    b. diastolic (always pathological).
    c. systolic (possibly benign).
    d. systolic (always pathological).

Match column A to column B.

Column A

15. _____ tough, fibrous, double-walled sac that surrounds and protects the heart

16. _____ thin layer of endothelial tissue that lines the inner surface of the heart chambers and valves

17. _____ reservoir for holding blood

18. _____ ensures smooth, friction-free movement of the heart muscle

19. _____ muscular pumping chamber

20. _____ muscular wall of the heart

Column B

a. pericardial fluid
b. ventricle
c. endocardium
d. myocardium
e. pericardium
f. atrium

21. Briefly relate the route of a blood cell from the liver to tissue in the body.

22. List the major risk factors of heart disease and stroke identified in the text.

SKILLS LABORATORY/CLINICAL SETTING

You are now ready for the clinical component of the cardiovascular system. The purpose of the clinical component is to practise the regional examination on a peer in the skills laboratory or a patient in the clinical setting and to achieve the following:

CLINICAL OBJECTIVES

1. Demonstrate knowledge of the symptoms related to the cardiovascular system by obtaining a regional health history from a peer or patient.

2. Correctly locate anatomic landmarks on the chest wall of a peer.

3. Using a grease pencil, and with peer's permission, outline borders of the heart, and label auscultatory areas on a peer's chest wall.

4. Demonstrate correct technique for inspection and palpation of the neck vessels.

5. Demonstrate correct techniques for inspection, palpation, and auscultation of the precordium.

6. Record the history and physical examination findings accurately, reach an assessment of the health state, and develop a plan of care.

INSTRUCTIONS

Gather your equipment. Wash your hands. Clean the stethoscope endpiece with an alcohol wipe. Practise the steps of the examination of the cardiovascular system on a peer or on a patient in the clinical area. Record your findings using the regional write-up sheet that follows. The front of the page is intended as a worksheet; the back of the page is intended for your narrative recording using the SOAP format.

NOTES

REGIONAL WRITE-UP—CARDIOVASCULAR SYSTEM

Date _____

Examiner _____

Patient _____ Age _____ Gender _____

Occupation _____

I. Health History

	No	Yes, explain
1. Any **chest pain** or tightness?		
2. Any **shortness of breath**?		
3. Use more than one pillow to sleep?		
4. Do you have a **cough**?		
5. Do you seem to **tire easily**?		
6. Facial skin ever turn blue or ashen?		
7. Any **swelling** of feet or legs?		
8. Awaken at night to urinate?		
9. Any past history of heart disease?		
10. Any family history of heart disease?		
11. Assess cardiac risk factors:		

II. Physical Examination

A. Carotid arteries
Inspect and palpate
Grade: R _____ L _____
(0 = absent, 1+ weak, 2+ normal, 3+ increased, 4+ bounding)

B. Jugular venous system
External jugular veins (circle one): < collapsed supine
meniscus visible at _____ bed elevated

Internal jugular venous pulsations
(circle one): < not visible
visible at _____ bed elevated

C. Precordium
Inspect and palpate
1. Skin colour and condition _____
2. Chest wall pulsations _____
3. Heave or lift _____
4. Apical impulse in the _____ at _____
   Size _____ Amplitude _____

D. Auscultation
1. Identify anatomic areas where you will listen.
2. Rate and rhythm _____
3. Identify S_1 and S_2 in diagram at right and note any
   variation:

S_1 S_2 S_1 S_2

S_1 _____

S_2 _____

4. Listen in systole and diastole:
   Extra heart sounds _____
   Systolic murmur _____
   Diastolic murmur _____

REGIONAL WRITE-UP—CARDIOVASCULAR SYSTEM

Summarize your findings using the SOAP format.

Subjective (Reason for seeking care, health history)

Objective (Physical examination findings)   Record findings using diagram

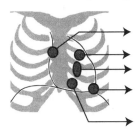

Assessment (Assessment of health state or problem, diagnosis)

Plan (Diagnostic evaluation, follow-up care, patient teaching)

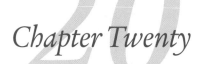

Chapter Twenty

Peripheral Vascular System and Lymphatic System

PURPOSE

This chapter helps you to learn the structure and function of the peripheral vascular system and the lymphatic system; to locate the peripheral pulse sites; to understand the rationale and methods of examination of the peripheral vascular and lymphatic systems; and to accurately record the assessment. At the end of this chapter you should be able to perform a complete assessment of the peripheral vascular and lymphatic systems.

READING ASSIGNMENT

Jarvis, *Physical Examination and Health Assessment,* 1st Canadian ed., Chapter 20, pp. 527–553.

_____

AUDIO-VISUAL ASSIGNMENT

Jarvis, *Physical Examination and Health Assessment DVD Series: Peripheral Vascular System and Lymphatic System*

_____

GLOSSARY

Study the following terms after completing the reading assignment. You should be able to cover the definition on the right and define the term out loud.

Allen test....................................determining the patency of the radial and ulnar arteries by compressing one artery site and observing return of skin colour as evidence of patency of the other artery

Aneurysm....................................defect or sac formed by dilation in artery wall due to atherosclerosis, trauma, or congenital defect

Arrhythmia................................variation from the heart's normal rhythm

Arteriosclerosis ....thickening and loss of elasticity of the arterial walls

Atherosclerosis ....plaques of fatty deposits formed in the inner layer (intima) of the arteries

Bradycardia ....slow heart rate, <50 beats per minute in the adult

Bruit...blowing, swooshing sound heard through a stethoscope when an artery is partially occluded

Cyanosis ....dusky blue mottling of the skin and mucous membranes due to excessive amount of reduced hemoglobin in the blood

Diastole ....the heart's filling phase

Homans' sign ....calf pain that occurs when the foot is sharply dorsiflexed (pushed up, toward the knee); may occur with deep vein thrombosis, phlebitis, Achilles tendinitis, or muscle injury

Ischemia ....deficiency of arterial blood to a body part, due to constriction or obstruction of a blood vessel

Lymphedema ....swelling of extremity due to obstructed lymph channel, nonpitting

Lymph nodes...............................small oval clumps of lymphatic tissue located at grouped intervals along lymphatic vessels

Pitting edema..............................indentation left after examiner depresses the skin over swollen edematous tissue

Profile sign ....viewing the finger from the side in order to detect early clubbing

Pulse ....pressure wave created by each heartbeat, palpable at body sites where the artery lies close to the skin and over a bone

Pulsus alternans ....regular rhythm, but force of pulse varies with alternating beats of large and small amplitude

Pulsus bigeminus ....irregular rhythm in which every other beat is premature; premature beats have weakened amplitude

Pulsus paradoxus ....beats have weaker amplitude with respiratory inspiration, stronger with expiration

Systole..the heart's pumping phase

Tachycardia ....rapid heart rate, >100 beats per minute in the adult

Thrombophlebitis........................inflammation of a vein associated with thrombus formation

Varicose vein ....dilated tortuous veins with incompetent valves

Ulcer...open skin lesion extending into dermis with sloughing of necrotic inflammatory tissue

STUDY GUIDE

After completing the reading assignment and the audio-visual assignment, you should be able to answer the following questions in the spaces provided.

1. Describe the structure and function of arteries and veins.

2. List the pulse sites accessible to examination.

3. Describe three mechanisms that help return venous blood to the heart.

4. Define the term *capacitance vessels* and explain its significance.

5. List the risk factors for venous stasis.

6. Describe the function of the lymphatic system.

7. Describe the function of the lymph nodes.

8. Name the related organs in the lymphatic system.

9. List the symptom areas to address during history-taking relating to the peripheral vascular system.

10. Fill in the grading scale for assessing the force of an arterial pulse: 0 = _____; 1+ _____; 2+ _____; 3+ _____; 4+ _____

11. List the steps in performing the modified Allen test.

12. List the skin characteristics expected with arterial insufficiency to the lower legs.

13. Compare the characteristics of leg ulcers associated with arterial insufficiency to ulcers with venous insufficiency.

14. Fill in the description of the grading scale for pitting edema:

1+ _____

2+ _____

3+ _____

4+ _____

15. Describe the technique for using the Doppler ultrasonic stethoscope to detect peripheral pulses.

16. Raynaud's phenomenon has associated progressive tricolour changes of the skin from _____

    to _____ and then to _____. State the mechanism for each of these colour changes.

Fill in the labels indicated on the following arteries and pulse sites.

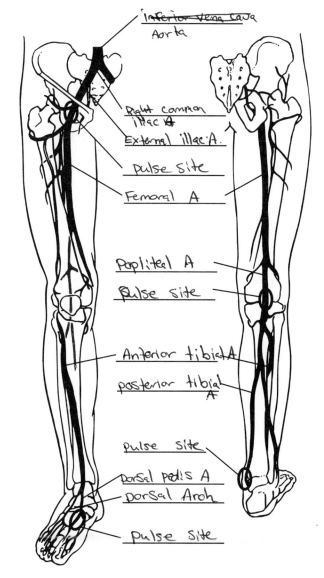

Inferior vena cava
Aorta

Right common iliac A
External iliac A.
Pulse site
Femoral A

Popliteal A
Pulse site

Anterior tibial A
posterior tibial A

Pulse site
Dorsal pedis A
Dorsal Arch
Pulse site

REVIEW QUESTIONS

This test is for you to check your own mastery of the content. Answers are provided in Appendix A.

1. A function of the venous system is:

   a. to hold more blood when blood volume increases.
   b. to conserve fluid and plasma proteins that leak out of the capillaries.
   c. to form a major part of the immune system that defends the body against disease.
   d. to absorb lipids from the intestinal tract.

2. The organs that aid the lymphatic system are:

   a. liver, lymph nodes, and stomach.
   b. pancreas, small intestine, and thymus.
   c. spleen, tonsils, and thymus.
   d. pancreas, spleen, and tonsils.

3. Ms. T. has come for a prenatal visit. She complains of dependent edema, varicosities in the legs, and hemorrhoids. The best response is:

   a. "If these symptoms persist, we will perform an amniocentesis."
   b. "If these symptoms persist, we will discuss having you hospitalized."
   c. "The symptoms are caused by the pressure of the growing uterus on the veins. They are usual conditions of pregnancy."
   d. "At this time, the symptoms are a minor inconvenience. You should learn to accept them."

4. A pulse with an amplitude of 3+ would be considered:

   a. bounding.
   b. increased.
   c. normal.
   d. weak.

5. Inspection of a person's right hand reveals a red, swollen area. To further assess for infection, you would palpate the:

   a. cervical node.
   b. axillary node.
   c. epitrochlear node.
   d. inguinal node.

6. In order to screen for deep vein thrombosis, you would:

   a. measure the circumference of the ankle.
   b. check the temperature with the palm of the hand.
   c. compress the dorsalis pedis pulse, looking for blood return.
   d. measure the widest point with a tape measure.

7. During the examination of the lower extremities, you are unable to palpate the popliteal pulse. You should:

   a. proceed with the examination. It is often impossible to palpate this pulse.
   b. refer the patient to a vascular surgeon for further evaluation.
   c. schedule the patient for a venogram.
   d. schedule the patient for an arteriogram.

8. While reviewing a medical record, a notation of 4+ edema of the right leg is noted. The best description of this type of edema is:

   a. mild pitting, no perceptible swelling of the leg.
   b. moderate pitting, indentation subsides rapidly.
   c. deep pitting, leg looks swollen.
   d. very deep pitting, indentation lasts a long time.

9. The examiner wishes to assess for arterial deficit in the lower extremities. After raising the legs 30 cm off the table and then having the person sit up and dangle the leg, the colour should return in:

   a. 5 seconds or less.
   b. 10 seconds or less.
   c. 15 seconds.
   d. 30 seconds.

10. A 54-year-old woman with five children has varicose veins of the lower extremities. Her most characteristic sign is:

    a. reduced arterial circulation.
    b. blanching, deathlike appearance of the extremities on elevation.
    c. loss of hair on feet and toes.
    d. dilated, tortuous, superficial bluish vessels.

11. Atrophic skin changes that occur with peripheral arterial insufficiency include:

    a. thin, shiny skin with loss of hair.
    b. brown discoloration.
    c. thick, leathery skin.
    d. slow-healing blisters on the skin.

12. Intermittent claudication is:

    a. muscular pain relieved by exercise.
    b. neurological pain relieved by exercise.
    c. muscular pain brought on by exercise.
    d. neurological pain brought on by exercise.

13. A known risk factor for venous ulcer development is:

    a. obesity.
    b. male gender.
    c. history of hypertension.
    d. daily aspirin therapy.

14. Brawny edema is:

    a. acute in onset.
    b. soft.
    c. nonpitting.
    d. associated with diminished pulses.

SKILLS LABORATORY/CLINICAL SETTING

You are now ready for the clinical component of the peripheral vascular system. The purpose of the clinical component is to practise the regional examination on a peer in the skills laboratory or a patient in the clinical setting and to achieve the following:

CLINICAL OBJECTIVES

1. Demonstrate knowledge of the symptoms related to the peripheral vascular system by obtaining a regional health history from a peer or patient.

2. Demonstrate palpation of peripheral arterial pulses (brachial, radial, femoral, popliteal, posterior tibial, dorsalis pedis) by assessing amplitude and symmetry, noting any signs of arterial insufficiency.

3. Demonstrate inspection and palpation of peripheral veins by noting any signs of venous insufficiency.

4. Demonstrate palpation of lymphatic system by identifying enlargement, clumping, or abnormal firmness of regional lymph nodes.

5. Demonstrate correct technique for performing the following additional tests when indicated: Allen test; Trendelenburg's test; manual compression test; Doppler ultrasonic stethoscope; computing the ankle–arm index.

6. Record the history and physical examination findings accurately, reach an assessment of the health state, and develop a plan of care.

INSTRUCTIONS

Gather your equipment. Wash your hands. Practise the steps of the examination of the peripheral vascular system on a peer or on a patient in the clinical setting, giving appropriate instructions as you proceed. Record your findings using the regional write-up sheets that follow. The first part is intended as a worksheet; the last page is intended for your narrative summary recording using the SOAP format. Note that the peripheral examination and cardiovascular examination usually are practised together.

NOTES

REGIONAL WRITE-UP—PERIPHERAL VASCULAR SYSTEM

Date _____

Examiner _____

Patient _____ Age _____ Gender _____

Occupation _____

I. Health History

	No	Yes, explain
1. Any leg **pain** (cramps)? Where?	_____	_____
2. Any **skin changes** in arms or legs?	_____	_____
3. Any sores or **lesions** in arms or legs?	_____	_____
4. Any **swelling** in the legs?	_____	_____
5. Any **swollen glands**? Where?	_____	_____
6. What medications are you taking?	_____	_____

II. Physical Examination

A. Inspection

1. The arms

   Inspect

   Colour of skin and nailbeds _____

   Symmetry _____

   Lesions _____

   Edema _____

   Clubbing _____

   Palpate _____

   Temperature _____

   Texture _____

   Capillary refill _____

   Locate and grade pulses (record on back)

   Check epitrochlear lymph node _____

   Modified Allen test (if indicated) _____

2. The legs

   Inspect

   Colour _____

   Hair distribution _____

   Venous pattern/varicosities _____

   Size _____

   Swelling/edema _____

   Atrophy _____

   If so, measure calf circumference in cm R _____   L _____

   Skin lesions or ulcers _____

   Palpate

   Temperature _____

   Tenderness _____

   Inguinal lymph nodes _____

   Locate and grade pulses (record on back)

   Check pretibial edema (grade if present) _____

   Auscultate for bruit (if indicated) _____

Jarvis, Luctkar-Flude: PHYSICAL EXAMINATION AND HEALTH ASSESSMENT, First Canadian Edition,
Student Laboratory Manual. Copyright © 2009 by Elsevier Canada, a division of Reed Elsevier Canada, Ltd. All rights rreserved.

REGIONAL WRITE-UP—PERIPHERAL VASCULAR SYSTEM

	Brachial	Radial	Femoral	Popliteal	D. pedis	P. tibial
R						
L						

0 = absent, 1+ = weak, 2+ = normal, 3+ = full, 4+ = bounding.

3. Additional tests
   Manual compression test _____
   Check colour change: elevate legs, then dangle; colour returns in _____ seconds
   Doppler ultrasonic stethoscope
      Locate pulse sites
      Ankle-brachial index (ABI)
      _____ ankle systolic pressure
      _____ = ____.____ or ____%
      _____ arm systolic pressure

REGIONAL WRITE-UP—PERIPHERAL VASCULAR SYSTEM

Summarize your findings using the SOAP format.

Subjective (Reason for seeking care, health history)

Objective (Physical examination findings)

Record pulses on diagram below

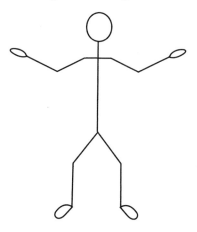

Assessment (Assessment of health state or problem, diagnosis)

Plan (Diagnostic evaluation, follow-up care, teaching)

NOTES

The Abdomen

PURPOSE

This chapter helps you to learn the structure and function of the abdominal organs; to know the location of the abdominal organs; to discriminate normal bowel sounds; to understand the rationale and methods of examination of the abdomen; and to accurately record the assessment. At the end of this chapter you should be able to perform a complete assessment of the abdomen.

READING ASSIGNMENT

Jarvis, *Physical Examination and Health Assessment,* 1st Canadian ed., Chapter 21, pp. 555–593.

AUDIO-VISUAL ASSIGNMENT

Jarvis, *Physical Examination and Health Assessment DVD Series: Abdomen*

GLOSSARY

Study the following terms after completing the reading assignment. You should be able to cover the definition on the right and define the term out loud.

Aneurysm....................................defect or sac formed by dilation in artery wall due to atherosclerosis, trauma, or congenital defect

Anorexia....................................loss of appetite for food

Ascites..abnormal accumulation of serous fluid within the peritoneal cavity, associated with congestive heart failure, cirrhosis, cancer, or portal hypertension

Borborygmi..............................loud gurgling bowel sounds signalling increased motility or hyperperistalsis; occur with early bowel obstruction, gastroenteritis, diarrhea

Bruit..blowing, swooshing sound heard through a stethoscope when an artery is partially occluded

Cecum..first or proximal part of large intestine

Cholecystitis ....inflammation of the gallbladder

Costal margin ....lower border of rib margin formed by the medial edges of the eighth, ninth, and tenth ribs

Costovertebral angle (CVA) ......angle formed by the twelfth rib and the vertebral column on the posterior thorax, overlying the kidney

Diastasis recti ....midline longitudinal ridge in the abdomen, a separation of abdominal rectus muscles

Dysphagia ....difficulty swallowing

Epigastrium ....name of abdominal region between the costal margins

Hepatomegaly ....abnormal enlargement of liver

Hernia ....abnormal protrusion of bowel through weakening in abdominal musculature

Inguinal ligament ....ligament extending from pubic bone to anterior superior iliac spine, forming lower border of abdomen

Linea alba ....midline tendinous seam joining the abdominal muscles

Paralytic ileus ....complete absence of peristaltic movement that may follow abdominal surgery or complete bowel obstruction

Peritoneal friction rub ....rough grating sound heard through the stethoscope over the site of peritoneal inflammation

Peritonitis ....inflammation of peritoneum

Pyloric stenosis ....congenital narrowing of pyloric sphincter, forming outflow obstruction of stomach

Pyrosis ....(heartburn) burning sensation in upper abdomen, due to reflux of gastric acid

Rectus abdominis muscle ....midline abdominal muscles extending from rib cage to pubic bone

Scaphoid ....abnormally sunken abdominal wall, as with malnutrition or underweight

Splenomegaly ....abnormal enlargement of spleen

Striae ....(linea albicantes) silvery white or pink scar tissue formed by stretching of abdominal skin, as with pregnancy or obesity

Suprapubic ....name of abdominal region just superior to pubic bone

Tympany ....high-pitched, musical, drumlike percussion note heard when percussing over the stomach and intestine

Umbilicus ....depression on the abdomen marking site of entry of umbilical cord

Viscera ....internal organs

STUDY GUIDE

After completing the reading assignment and the audio-visual assignment, you should be able to answer the following questions in the spaces provided.

1. Draw a picture of the borders of the abdomen. Draw in the organs.

2. Name the organs that are normally palpable in the abdomen.

3. Describe the proper positioning and preparation of the patient for the examination.

4. State the rationale for performing auscultation of the abdomen before palpation or percussion.

5. Discuss inspection of the abdomen, including findings that should be noted.

6. Describe the procedure for auscultation of bowel sounds.

7. Differentiate the following abdominal sounds: normal, hyperactive, and hypoactive bowel sounds, succession splash, bruit.

8. Identify and give the rationale for each of the percussion notes heard over the abdomen.

   a. List four conditions that may alter normal percussion notes.

9. Describe the procedure for percussing the liver span and the spleen.

10. Describe these manoeuvres and discuss their significance: fluid wave test, shifting dullness.

11. Differentiate between light and deep palpation, and explain the purpose of each.

   a. List two abnormalities that may be detected by light palpation and two detected by deep palpation.

12. Contrast rigidity with voluntary guarding.

13. Contrast visceral pain and somatic (parietal) pain.

14. Describe rebound tenderness.

15. Describe palpation of the liver, spleen, and kidney.

16. Distinguish abdominal wall masses from intra-abdominal masses.

17. Describe the procedure and rationale for determining costovertebral angle (CVA) tenderness.

18. Describe the expected examination findings of the abdomen in each of the following conditions:

Obesity _____

Gaseous distention _____

Tumour _____

Pregnancy _____

Ascites _____

Enlarged liver _____

Enlarged spleen _____

Distended bladder _____

Appendicitis _____

Fill in the labels indicated on the following illustrations.

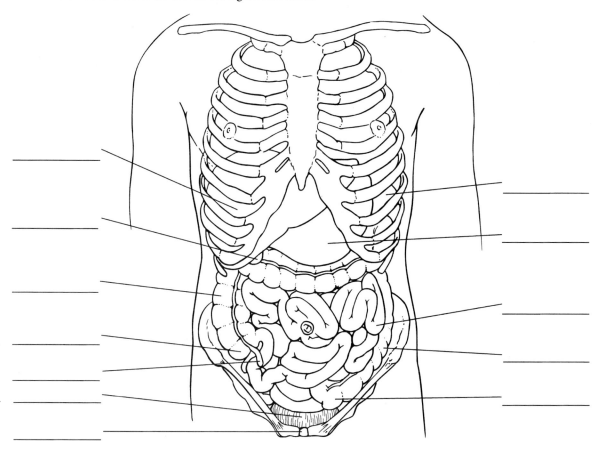

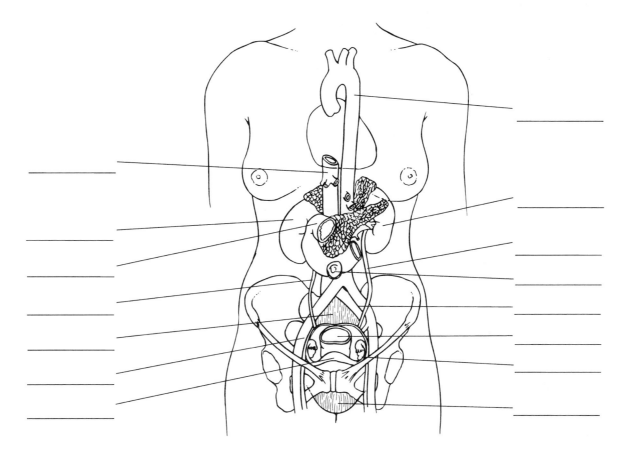

REVIEW QUESTIONS

This test is for you to check your own mastery of the content. Answers are provided in Appendix A.

1. Select the sequence of techniques used during an examination of the abdomen.

   a. percussion, inspection, palpation, auscultation
   b. inspection, palpation, percussion, auscultation
   c. inspection, auscultation, percussion, palpation
   d. auscultation, inspection, palpation, percussion

2. Which of the following may be noted through inspection of the abdomen?

   a. fluid waves and abdominal contour
   b. umbilical eversion and Murphy's sign
   c. venous pattern, peristaltic waves, and abdominal contour
   d. peritoneal irritation, general tympany, and peristaltic waves

3. Right upper quadrant tenderness may indicate pathology in the:

   a. liver, pancreas, or ascending colon.
   b. liver and stomach.
   c. sigmoid colon, spleen, or rectum.
   d. appendix or ileocecal valve.

4. Hyperactive bowel sounds are:

   a. high-pitched.
   b. rushing.
   c. tinkling.
   d. all of the above.

5. The absence of bowel sounds is established after listening for:

   a. 1 full minute.
   b. 3 full minutes.
   c. 5 full minutes.
   d. none of the above.

6. Auscultation of the abdomen may reveal bruits of the _____ arteries.

   a. aortic, renal, iliac, and femoral
   b. jugular, aortic, carotid, and femoral
   c. pulmonic, aortic, and portal
   d. renal, iliac, internal jugular, and basilic

7. The range of normal liver span in the right midclavicular line in the adult is:

   a. 2–6 cm.
   b. 4–8 cm.
   c. 8–14 cm.
   d. 6–12 cm.

8. The left upper quadrant (LUQ) contains the:

   a. liver.
   b. appendix.
   c. left ovary.
   d. spleen.

9. Striae, which occur when the elastic fibres in the reticular layer of the skin are broken following rapid or prolonged stretching, have a distinct colour when of long duration. This colour is:

   a. pink.
   b. blue.
   c. purple-blue.
   d. silvery white.

10. Auscultation of the abdomen is begun in the right lower quadrant (RLQ) because:

    a. bowel sounds are always normally present here.
    b. peristalsis through the descending colon is usually active.
    c. this is the location of the pyloric sphincter.
    d. vascular sounds are best heard in this area.

11. A dull percussion note forward of the left midaxillary line is:

    a. normal, an expected finding during splenic percussion.
    b. expected between the eighth and twelfth ribs.
    c. found if the examination follows a large meal.
    d. indicative of splenic enlargement.

12. Shifting dullness is a test for:

    a. ascites.
    b. splenic enlargement.
    c. inflammation of the kidney.
    d. hepatomegaly.

13. Tenderness during abdominal palpation is expected when palpating:

    a. the liver edge.
    b. the spleen.
    c. the sigmoid colon.
    d. the kidneys.

14. Murphy's sign is best described as:

    a. the pain felt when the hand of the examiner is rapidly removed from an inflamed appendix.
    b. pain felt when taking a deep breath when the examiner's fingers are on the approximate location of the inflamed gallbladder.
    c. a sharp pain felt by the patient when one hand of the examiner is used to thump the other at the costovertebral angle.
    d. not a valid examination technique.

SKILLS LABORATORY/CLINICAL SETTING

You are now ready for the clinical component of the abdominal system. The purpose of the clinical component is to practise the regional examination on a peer in the skills laboratory or a patient in the clinical setting and to achieve the following:

CLINICAL OBJECTIVES

1. Demonstrate knowledge of the symptoms related to the abdominal system by obtaining a regional health history from a peer or patient.

2. Demonstrate inspection of the abdomen by assessing skin condition, symmetry, contour, pulsation, umbilicus, and nutritional state.

3. Demonstrate auscultation of the abdomen by assessing characteristics of bowel sounds and by screening for bruits.

4. Demonstrate percussion of the abdomen by identifying the predominant percussion note, determining liver span, and noting borders of spleen.

5. Demonstrate light palpation by assessing muscular resistance, tenderness, and any masses.

6. Demonstrate deep palpation by assessing for any masses; the liver, spleen, kidneys, and aorta; and any CVA or rebound tenderness.

7. Demonstrate correct technique of performing the following additional tests when indicated: inspiratory arrest; iliopsoas muscle test; and obturator test.

8. Record the history and physical examination findings accurately, reach an assessment of the health state, and develop a plan of care.

INSTRUCTIONS

Gather your equipment. Wash your hands. Assess the patient's comfort before starting. Practise the steps of the examination on a peer or a patient in the clinical setting, giving appropriate instructions as you proceed. Record your findings using the regional write-up sheets that follow. The front of the page is intended as a worksheet; the back of the page is intended for your narrative summary recording using the SOAP format.

NOTES

REGIONAL WRITE-UP—ABDOMEN

Date _____

Examiner _____

Patient _____ Age _____ Gender _____

Occupation _____

I. Health History

	No	Yes, explain
1. Any change in **appetite**? Loss?		
2. Any difficulty **swallowing**?		
3. Any foods you **cannot tolerate**?		
4. Any **abdominal pain**?		
5. Any **nausea or vomiting**?		
6. How often are **bowel movements**?		
7. Any past history of **GI disease**?		
8. What **medications** are you taking?		

9. Tell me all food you ate in the last **24 hours,** starting with:

breakfast   snack   lunch   snack   dinner   snack

II. Physical Examination

A. Inspection
Contour of abdomen _____
General symmetry _____
Skin colour and condition _____
Pulsation or movement _____
Umbilicus _____
Hair distribution _____
State of hydration and nutrition _____
Person's facial expression and position in bed _____

B. Auscultation
Bowel sounds _____
Note any vascular sounds _____

C. Percussion
Percuss in all four quadrants _____
Percuss borders of liver span in R MCL _____ cm _____
Percuss spleen _____
If suspect ascites, test for fluid wave and shifting dullness _____

D. Palpation
Light palpation in all four quadrants
  Muscle wall _____
  Tenderness _____
  Enlarged organs _____
  Masses _____

Deep palpation in all four quadrants
  Masses _____
  Contour of liver _____
  Spleen _____
  Kidneys _____
  Aorta _____
  Rebound tenderness _____
  CVA tenderness _____
  E. Additional tests, if indicated

REGIONAL WRITE-UP—ABDOMEN

Summarize your findings using the SOAP format.

Subjective (Reason for seeking care, health history)

Objective (Physical examination findings)
Record findings on diagram

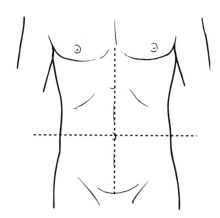

Assessment (Assessment of health state or problem, diagnosis)

Plan (Diagnostic evaluation, follow-up care, teaching)

Chapter Twenty-Two

Musculoskeletal System

PURPOSE

This chapter helps you to learn the structure and function of the various joints in the body; to know their normal ranges of motion; to position the patient comfortably during the examination; to understand the rationale and methods of examination of the musculoskeletal system; to assess functional ability; and to accurately record the assessment. At the end of this chapter you should be able to perform a complete assessment of the musculoskeletal system.

READING ASSIGNMENT

Jarvis, *Physical Examination and Health Assessment,* 1st Canadian ed., Chapter 22, pp. 595–652.

AUDIO-VISUAL ASSIGNMENT

Jarvis, *Physical Examination and Health Assessment DVD Series: Musculoskeletal System*

GLOSSARY

Study the following terms after completing the reading assignment. You should be able to cover the definition on the right and define the term out loud.

Abduction ....moving a body part away from an axis or the median line

Adduction ....moving a body part toward the centre or toward the median line

Ankylosis....................................immobility, consolidation, and fixation of a joint because of disease, injury, or surgery; most often due to chronic rheumatoid arthritis

Ataxia..inability to perform coordinated movements

Bursa...enclosed sac filled with viscous fluid located in joint areas of potential friction

Circumduction ....moving the arm in a circle around the shoulder

Crepitation.................................dry crackling sound or sensation due to grating of the ends of damaged bone

Dorsal ....directed toward or located on the surface

Dupuytren's contracture ....flexion contractures of the fingers due to chronic hyperplasia of the palmar fascia

Eversion ....moving the sole of the foot outward at the ankle

Extension.....................................straightening a limb at a joint

Flexion ....bending a limb at a joint

Ganglion......................................round, cystic, nontender nodule overlying a tendon sheath or joint capsule, usually on dorsum of wrist

Hallux valgus ....lateral or outward deviation of the great toe

Inversion ....moving the sole of the foot inward at the ankle

Kyphosis.....................................outward or convex curvature of the thoracic spine, hunchback

Ligament ....fibrous bands running directly from one bone to another bone that strengthen the joint

Lordosis......................................inward or concave curvature of the lumbar spine

Nucleus pulposus ....centre of the intervertebral disc

Olecranon process......................bony projection of the ulna at the elbow

Patella ....kneecap

Plantar ....surface of the sole of the foot

Pronation ....turning the forearm so that the palm is down

Protraction ....moving a body part forward and parallel to the ground

Range of motion (ROM) ....extent of movement of a joint

Retraction ....moving a body part backward and parallel to the ground

Rheumatoid arthritis ....chronic systemic inflammatory disease of joints and surrounding connective tissue

Sciatica ....nerve pain along the course of the sciatic nerve that travels down from the back or thigh through the leg and into the foot

Scoliosis......................................S-shaped curvature of the thoracic spine

Supination ....turning the forearm so that the palm is up

Talipes equinovarus...................(clubfoot) congenital deformity of the foot in which it is plantar flexed and inverted

Tendon...strong fibrous cord that attaches a skeletal muscle to a bone

Torticollis ....(wryneck) contraction of the cervical neck muscles, producing torsion of the neck

STUDY GUIDE

After completing the reading assignment and the audio-visual assignment, you should be able to answer the following questions in the spaces provided.

1. List four signs that suggest acute inflammation in a joint.

2. Differentiate the following:

   Dislocation

   Subluxation

   Contracture

   Ankylosis

3. Describe the correct method for use of the goniometer.

4. Differentiate testing of active range of motion versus passive range of motion.

5. State the expected range of degrees of flexion and extension of the following joints:

   Elbow

   Wrist

   Fingers (at metacarpophalangeal joints)

6. State the expected range of degrees of flexion and extension of the following joints:

   Hip

   Knee

   Ankle

7. Explain the method for measuring leg length.

8. Describe the Ortolani manoeuvre for checking an infant's hips.

9. State four landmarks to note when checking an adolescent for scoliosis.

10. When performing a functional assessment for an older adult, state the common adaptations the aging person makes when attempting these manoeuvres:

Walking _____

Climbing up stairs _____

Walking down stairs _____

Picking up object from floor _____

Rising up from sitting in chair _____

Rising up from lying in bed _____

11. Describe the symptoms and signs in carpal tunnel syndrome.

Name and describe two techniques of examination for the syndrome.

12. Draw and describe swan-neck deformity and boutonnière deformity.

13. Contrast Bouchard's nodes with Heberden's nodes.

14. Contrast syndactyly and polydactyly.

Fill in the labels indicated on the following illustrations.

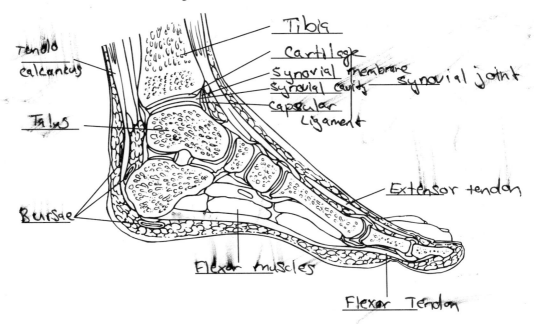

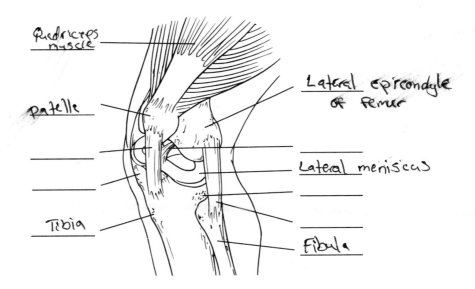

REVIEW QUESTIONS

This test is for you to check your own mastery of the content. Answers are provided in Appendix A.

1. During an assessment of the spine, the patient would be asked to:

   a. adduct and extend.
   b. supinate, evert, and retract.
   c. extend, adduct, invert, and rotate.
   d. flex, extend, abduct, and rotate.

2. Pronation and supination of the hand and forearm are the result of the articulation of the:

   a. scapula and clavicle.
   b. radius and ulna.
   c. patella and condyle of fibula.
   d. femur and acetabulum.

3. Anterior and posterior stability is provided to the knee joint by the:

   a. medial and lateral menisci.
   b. patellar tendon and ligament.
   c. medial collateral ligament and quadriceps muscle.
   d. anterior and posterior cruciate ligaments.

4. A 70-year-old woman has come for a health examination. Which of the following is a common age-related change in the curvature of the spinal column?

   a. lordosis
   b. scoliosis
   c. kyphosis
   d. lateral scoliosis

5. The timing of joint pain may assist the examiner in determining the cause. The joint pain associated with rheumatic fever would:

   a. be worse in the morning.
   b. be worse later in the day.
   c. be worse in the morning but improve during the day.
   d. occur 10 to 14 days after an untreated sore throat.

6. Examination of the shoulder includes four motions. These are:

   a. forward flexion, internal rotation, abduction, and external rotation.
   b. abduction, adduction, pronation, and supination.
   c. circumduction, inversion, eversion, and rotation.
   d. elevation, retraction, protraction, and circumduction.

7. The bulge sign is a test for:

   a. swelling in the suprapatellar pouch.
   b. carpal tunnel syndrome.
   c. Heberden's nodes.
   d. olecranon bursa inflammation.

8. The examiner is going to measure the patient's legs for length discrepancy. The normal finding would be:

   a. no difference in measurements.
   b. 0.5 cm difference.
   c. within 1 cm of each other.
   d. 2 cm difference.

9. A two-year-old child has been brought to the clinic for a health examination. A common finding would be:

   a. kyphosis.
   b. lordosis.
   c. scoliosis.
   d. no deviation is normal.

10. Briefly describe the functions of the musculoskeletal system.

Match column A with column B.

Column A—Movement	Column B—Description
11. _____ Flexion	a. turning the forearm so that the palm is up
12. _____ Extension	b. bending a limb at a joint
13. _____ Abduction	c. lowering a body part
14. _____ Adduction	d. turning the forearm so that the palm is down
15. _____ Pronation	e. straightening a limb at a joint
16. _____ Supination	f. raising a body part
17. _____ Circumduction	g. moving a limb away from the midline of the body
18. _____ Inversion	h. moving a body part backward and parallel to the ground
19. _____ Eversion	i. moving a limb toward the midline of the body
20. _____ Rotation	j. moving the arm in a circle around the shoulder
21. _____ Protraction	k. moving the sole of the foot outward at the ankle
22. _____ Retraction	l. moving a body part forward and parallel to the ground
23. _____ Elevation	m. moving the sole of the foot inward at the ankle
24. _____ Depression	n. moving the head around a central axis

SKILLS LABORATORY/CLINICAL SETTING

You are now ready for the clinical component of the musculoskeletal system. The purpose of the clinical component is to practise the regional examination on a peer in the skills laboratory or a patient in the clinical setting and to achieve the following:

CLINICAL OBJECTIVES

1. Demonstrate knowledge of the symptoms related to the musculoskeletal system by obtaining a regional health history from a peer or patient.

2. Demonstrate inspection and palpation of the musculoskeletal system by assessing the muscles, bones, and joints for size, symmetry, swelling, nodules, deformities, atrophy, and active range of motion.

3. Assess the person's ability to carry out functional activities of daily living.

4. Record the history and physical examination findings accurately, reach an assessment about the health state, and develop a plan of care.

INSTRUCTIONS

Gather your equipment. Wash your hands. Practise the steps of the examination on a peer or a patient in the clinical setting, giving appropriate instructions as you proceed, and maintaining the safety of the person during movement. Record your findings using the regional write-up sheet that follows. The first section is intended as a worksheet; the last page is intended for your narrative summary recording using the SOAP format.

Note the student performance checklist that follows the regional write-up sheet. It lists the essential behaviours you should display as an examiner, and it may be used by your clinical instructor to evaluate your clinical musculoskeletal examination.

NOTES

REGIONAL WRITE-UP—MUSCULOSKELETAL SYSTEM

Date _____

Examiner _____

Patient _____ Age _____ Gender _____

Occupation _____

I. Health History

	No	Yes, explain

1. Any **pain** in the joints?
2. Any **stiffness** in the joints?
3. Any **swelling, heat, redness** in joints?
4. Any **limitation of movement**?
5. Any **muscle pain** or cramping?
6. Any **deformity** of bone or joint?
7. Any **accidents or trauma** to bones?
8. Ever had **back pain**?
9. Any problems with the activities of daily living: bathing, toileting, dressing, grooming, eating, mobility, communicating?

II. Physical Examination

A. Cervical spine
1. Inspect size, contour _____ Mass or deformity _____
2. Palpate for temperature _____ Pain _____
   Swelling or mass _____
3. Active range of motion
   Flexion _____ Extension _____
   Lateral bending right _____ Left _____
   Right rotation _____ Left _____

B. Shoulders
1. Inspect size, contour _____ Colour, swelling _____
   Mass or deformity _____
2. Palpate for temperature _____ Pain _____
   Swelling or mass _____
3. Active range of motion
   Flexion _____ Extension _____
   Abduction _____ Adduction _____
   Internal rotation _____ External rotation _____

C. Elbows

1. Inspect for size, contour _____ Colour, swelling _____
   Mass or deformity _____
2. Palpate for temperature _____ Pain _____
   Swelling or mass _____
3. Active range of motion
   Flexion _____ Extension _____
   Pronation _____ Supination _____

D. Wrists and hands

1. Inspect for size, contour _____ Colour, swelling _____
   Mass or deformity _____
2. Palpate for temperature _____ Pain _____
   Swelling or mass _____
3. Active range of motion
   Wrist extension _____ Flexion _____
   Finger extension _____ Flexion _____
   Ulnar deviation _____ Radial deviation _____
   Fingers spread _____ Make fist _____
   Touch thumb to each finger _____

E. Hips

1. Inspect size, contour _____ Colour, swelling _____
   Mass or deformity _____
2. Palpate for temperature _____ Pain _____
   Swelling or mass _____
3. Active range of motion
   Extension _____ Flexion _____
   External rotation _____ Internal rotation _____
   Abduction _____ Adduction _____

F. Knees

1. Inspect size, contour _____ Colour, swelling _____
   Mass or deformity _____
2. Palpate for temperature _____ Pain _____
   Swelling or mass _____
3. Active range of motion
   Flexion _____ Extension _____
   Walk _____ Shallow knee bend _____

G. Ankles and feet

1. Inspect for size, contour _____ Colour, swelling _____
   Mass or deformity _____
2. Palpate for temperature _____ Pain _____
   Swelling or mass _____
3. Active range of motion
   Dorsiflexion _____ Plantar flexion _____
   Inversion _____ Eversion _____

H. Spine

    1. Inspect for straight spinous processes _____

       Equal horizontal positions for shoulders, scapulae, iliac crests, gluteal folds _____

       Equal spaces between arms and lateral thorax _____

       Knees and feet align with trunk, point forward _____

       From side note curvature: cervical, thoracic, lumbar _____

    2. Palpate spinous processes

    3. Active range of motion

       Flexion _____ Extension _____

       Lateral bending right _____ Left _____

       Rotation right _____ Left _____

I. Functional assessment (if indicated)

    Walk (with shoes on)

    Climb up stairs

    Walk down stairs

    Pick up object from floor

    Rise up from sitting in chair

    Rise up from lying in bed

REGIONAL WRITE-UP—MUSCULOSKELETAL SYSTEM

Summarize your findings using the SOAP format.

Subjective (Reason for seeking care, health history)

Objective (Physical examination findings)

Assessment (Assessment of health state or problem, diagnosis)

Plan (Diagnostic evaluation, follow-up care, patient teaching)

STUDENT COMPETENCY CHECKLIST

MUSCULOSKELETAL SYSTEM—ESSENTIAL BEHAVIOURS

	Yes	No	Comments
Obtain relevant history, functional and self-care assessments			
Gather equipment			
Tape measure			
Goniometer			
Skin marking pen			
Light if needed			
Provide privacy			
Wash hands			
Observe for symmetry			
Inspect each joint for: Size			
Contour			
Range of motion/limitation			
Inspect skin and tissue over joints for: Colour			
Swelling			
Masses			
Deformity			
Palpate each joint for: Heat			
Tenderness			
Swelling			
Masses			

	Yes	No	Comments
Test ROM			
Grade muscle strength			
Record findings including notations regarding specific joints			
Temporomandibular			
Cervical spine			
Shoulders			
Elbow			
Wrist			
Hand			
Hip			
Knee			
Ballottement test			
McMurray's test			
Ankle			
Foot			
Document findings			

Chapter Twenty-Three

Neurological System

PURPOSE

This chapter helps you to learn the structure and function of the components of the neurological system, including the cranial nerves, cerebellar system, motor system, sensory system, and reflexes; to understand the rationale and methods of examination of the neurological system; and to accurately record the assessment. Together with the mental status assessment presented in Chapter 6, you should be able to perform a complete assessment of the neurological system, at the end of this chapter.

READING ASSIGNMENT

Jarvis, *Physical Examination and Health Assessment,* 1st Canadian ed., Chapter 23, pp. 653–710.

AUDIO-VISUAL ASSIGNMENT

Jarvis, *Physical Examination and Health Assessment DVD Series: Neurologic: Cranial Nerves and Sensory System; Neurologic: Motor System and Reflexes*

GLOSSARY

Study the following terms after completing the reading assignment. You should be able to cover the definition on the right and define the term out loud.

Agnosia ....loss of ability to recognize importance of sensory impressions

Agraphia ....loss of ability to express thoughts in writing

Amnesia ....loss of memory

Analgesia ....loss of pain sensation

Aphasia ....loss of power of expression by speech, writing, or signs, or of comprehension of spoken or written language

Apraxia ....loss of ability to perform purposeful movements in the absence of sensory or motor damage; for example, inability to use objects correctly

Ataxia..inability to perform coordinated movements

Athetosis.......................................bizarre, slow, twisting, writhing movement, resembling a snake or worm

Chorea..sudden, rapid, jerky, purposeless movement involving limbs, trunk, or face

Clonus...rapidly alternating involuntary contraction and relaxation of a muscle in response to sudden stretch

Coma..state of profound unconsciousness from which person cannot be aroused

Decerebrate rigidity...................arms stiffly extended, adducted, internally rotated; legs stiffly extended, plantar flexed

Decorticate rigidity...................arms adducted and flexed, wrists and fingers flexed; legs extended, internally rotated, plantar flexed

Dysarthria..................................imperfect articulation of speech due to problems of muscular control resulting from central or peripheral nervous system damage

Dysphasia...................................impairment in speech consisting of lack of coordination and inability to arrange words in their proper order

Extinction..................................disappearance of conditioned response

Fasciculation..............................rapid continuous twitching of resting muscle without movement of limb

Flaccidity...................................loss of muscle tone, limp

Graphesthesia.............................ability to "read" a number by having it traced on the skin

Hemiplegia.................................loss of motor power (paralysis) on one side of the body, usually caused by a cerebrovascular accident; paralysis occurs on the side opposite the lesion

Lower motor neuron...................motor neuron in the peripheral nervous system with its nerve fibre extending out to the muscle and only its cell body in the central nervous system

Myoclonus..................................rapid sudden jerk of a muscle

Nuchal rigidity...........................stiffness in cervical neck area

Nystagmus..................................back-and-forth oscillation of the eyes

Opisthotonos..............................prolonged arching of back, with head and heels bent backward, and meningeal irritation

Paralysis.....................................decrease or loss of motor function due to problem with motor nerve or muscle fibres

Paraplegia..................................impairment or loss of motor or sensory function, or both, in the lower half of the body

Paresthesia.................................abnormal sensation; that is, burning, numbness, tingling, prickling, or a crawling skin sensation

Point localization......................ability of the person to discriminate exactly where on the body the skin has been touched

Proprioception..........................sensory information concerning body movements and position of the body in space

Spasticity..................................continuous resistance to stretching by a muscle due to abnormally increased tension, with increased deep tendon reflexes

Stereognosis.............................ability to recognize objects by feeling their forms, sizes, and weights while the eyes are closed

Tic..repetitive twitching of a muscle group at inappropriate times; for example, wink, grimace

Tremor......................................involuntary contraction of opposing muscle groups resulting in rhythmic movement of one or more joints

Two-point discrimination.........ability to distinguish the separation of two simultaneous pinpricks on the skin

Upper motor neuron.................nerve located entirely within the central nervous system

STUDY GUIDE

After completing the reading assignment and the audio-visual assignment, you should be able to answer the following questions in the spaces provided.

1. List the major function(s) of the following components of the central nervous system:

Cerebral cortex—frontal lobe _____

Cerebral cortex—parietal lobe _____

Cerebral cortex—temporal lobe _____

Cerebral cortex—Wernicke's area _____

Cerebral cortex—Broca's area _____

Basal ganglia _____

Thalamus _____

Hypothalamus _____

Cerebellum _____

Midbrain _____

Pons _____

Medulla _____

Spinal cord _____

2. List the primary sensations mediated by the two major sensory pathways of the CNS.

3. Describe three major motor pathways in the CNS, including the type of movements mediated by each.

4. Differentiate an upper motor neuron from a lower motor neuron.

5. List the five components of a deep tendon reflex arc.

6. List the major symptom areas to assess when collecting a health history for the neurological system.

7. List the method of testing for each of the 12 cranial nerves.   CN-2-7

8. List and describe three tests of cerebellar function.

9. Describe the method of testing the sensory system for pain, temperature, touch, vibration, and position.

10. Define the four-point grading scale for deep tendon reflexes.

11. State the vertebral level whose intactness is assessed when eliciting each of these reflexes:

Biceps reflex _____

Triceps reflex _____

Brachioradialis reflex _____

Quadriceps reflex _____

Achilles reflex _____

12. List the components of the neurological recheck examination that are performed routinely on hospitalized persons being monitored for neurological deficit.

13. List the three areas of assessment on the Glasgow Coma Scale.

14. Describe the gait patterns of the following abnormal gaits:

Spastic hemiparesis

Cerebellar ataxia

Parkinsonian

Scissors

Steppage

Waddling

15. State the type of reflex response you would expect to see with an upper motor neuron lesion versus a lower motor neuron lesion.

16. Describe the method of testing the type of reflexes that are also termed *frontal release signs.*

Notes

Fill in the labels indicated on the following illustrations.

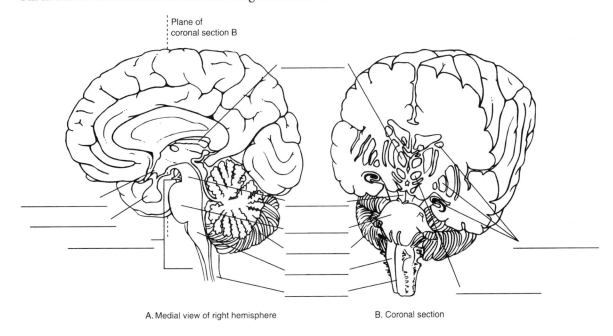

A. Medial view of right hemisphere

B. Coronal section

CONTENTS OF THE CENTRAL NERVOUS SYSTEM

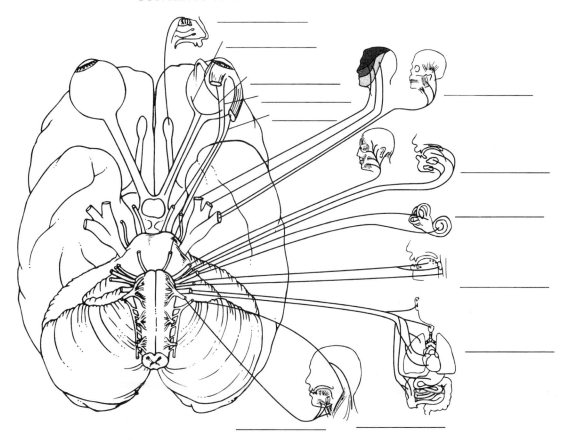

Fill in the name of each cranial nerve, then write S (sensory), M (Motor), or MX (mixed).

REVIEW QUESTIONS

This test is for you to check your own mastery of the content. The answers are provided in Appendix A.

1. The medical record indicates that a person has an injury to Broca's area. When meeting this person you expect:

   a. difficulty speaking.
   b. receptive aphasia.
   c. visual disturbances.
   d. emotional lability.

2. The control of body temperature is located in:

   a. Wernicke's area.
   b. the thalamus.
   c. the cerebellum.
   d. the hypothalamus.

3. To test for stereognosis, you would:

   a. have the person close his or her eyes, then raise the person's arm and ask the person to describe its location.
   b. touch the person with a tuning fork.
   c. place a coin in the person's hand and ask him or her to identify it.
   d. touch the person with a cold object.

4. During the examination of an infant, use a cotton-tipped applicator to stimulate the anal sphincter. The absence of a response suggests a lesion of:

   a. L2.
   b. T12.
   c. S2.
   d. C5.

5. During a neurological examination, the tendon reflex fails to appear. Before striking the tendon again, the examiner might use the technique of:

   a. two-point discrimination.
   b. reinforcement.
   c. vibration.
   d. graphesthesia.

6. Cerebellar function is assessed by which of the following tests?

   a. muscle size and strength
   b. cranial nerve examination
   c. coordination—hop on one foot
   d. spinothalamic test

7. To elicit a Babinski reflex:

   a. gently tap the Achilles tendon.
   b. stroke the lateral aspect of the sole of the foot from heel to the ball.
   c. present a noxious odour to a person.
   d. observe the person walking heel to toe.

8. A positive Babinski sign is:

   a. dorsiflexion of the big toe and fanning of all toes.
   b. plantar flexion of the big toe with a fanning of all toes.
   c. the expected response in healthy adults.
   d. withdrawal of the stimulated extremity from the stimulus.

9. The cremasteric response:

   a. is positive when disease of the pyramidal tract is present.
   b. is positive when the ipsilateral testicle elevates upon stroking of the inner aspect of the thigh.
   c. is a reflex of the receptors in the muscles of the abdomen.
   d. is not a valid neurological examination.

10. To examine for the function of the trigeminal nerve in an infant, you would:

   a. startle the baby.
   b. hold an object within the child's line of vision.
   c. pinch the nose of the child.
   d. offer the baby a bottle.

11. Senile tremors may resemble parkinsonism, except that senile tremors do not include:

   a. nodding the head as if responding yes or no.
   b. rigidity and weakness of voluntary movement.
   c. tremor of the hands.
   d. tongue protrusion.

12. People who have Parkinson's disease usually have which of the following characteristic styles of speech?

   a. a garbled manner
   b. loud, urgent
   c. slow, monotonous
   d. word confusion

Match column A with column B.

Column A—Cranial Nerve	Column B—Function
13. ___F___ Olfactory	a. movement of the tongue
14. _____ Optic	b. vision
15. _____ Oculomotor	c. lateral movement of the eyes
16. _____ Trochlear	d. hearing and equilibrium
17. _____ Trigeminal	e. talking, swallowing, carotid sinus, and carotid reflex
18. _____ Abducens	f. smell
19. _____ Facial	g. extraocular movement, pupil constriction, down and inward movement of the eye
20. _____ Acoustic	h. mastication and sensation of face, scalp, cornea
21. _____ Glossopharyngeal	i. phonation, swallowing, taste in the posterior third of tongue
22. _____ Vagus	j. movement of trapezius and sternomastoid muscles
23. _____ Spinal	k. down and inward movement of the eye
24. _____ Hypoglossal	l. taste in the anterior two thirds of tongue, closing of the eyes

SKILLS LABORATORY/CLINICAL SETTING

You are now ready for the clinical component of the neurological system. The purpose of the clinical component is to practise the regional examination on a peer in the skills laboratory or a patient in the clinical setting and to achieve the following:

CLINICAL OBJECTIVES

1. Demonstrate knowledge of the symptoms related to the neurological system by obtaining a regional health history from a peer or patient.

2. Demonstrate examination of the neurological system by assessing the cranial nerves, cerebellar function, sensory system, motor system, and deep tendon reflexes.

3. Record the history and physical examination findings accurately, reach an assessment of the health state, and develop a plan of care.

INSTRUCTIONS

Gather all equipment for a complete neurological examination. Wash your hands. Practise the steps of the examination on a peer or a patient in the clinical setting, giving appropriate instructions as you proceed. Record your findings using the regional write-up sheet that follows. The first section is intended as a worksheet; the last page is intended for your narrative summary recording using the SOAP format.

NOTES

REGIONAL WRITE-UP—NEUROLOGICAL SYSTEM

Date _____

Examiner _____

Patient _____ Age _____ Gender _____

Occupation _____

I. Health History

	No	Yes, explain
1. Any unusual frequent or unusually severe **headaches**?	_____	_____
2. Ever had any **head injury**?	_____	_____
3. Ever feel **dizziness**?	_____	_____
4. Ever had any **convulsions**?	_____	_____
5. Any **tremors** in hands or face?	_____	_____
6. Any **weakness** in any body part?	_____	_____
7. Any problem with **coordination**?	_____	_____
8. Any **numbness or tingling**?	_____	_____
9. Any problem **swallowing**?	_____	_____
10. Any problem **speaking**?	_____	_____
11. Past history of stroke, spinal cord injury, meningitis, congenital defect, alcoholism?	_____	_____
12. Any environmental or occupational hazards, e.g., insecticides?	_____	_____

II. Physical Examination

A. Cranial nerves

I _____

II _____

III, IV, VI _____

V _____

VII _____

VIII _____

IX, X _____

XI _____

XII _____

B. Motor system

1. Muscles

   Size, strength, tone _____

   Involuntary movements _____

2. Cerebellar function

   Gait _____

   Romberg test _____

   Rapid alternative movements _____

   Finger-to-finger test _____

   Finger-to-nose test _____

   Heel-to-shin test _____

C. Sensory system

1. Spinothalamic tract
   Pain _____
   Temperature _____
   Light touch _____
2. Posterior column tract
   Vibration _____
   Position (kinesthesia) _____
   Tactile discrimination _____
     Stereognosis _____
     Graphesthesia _____
     Two-point discrimination _____

D. Reflexes

	Bi	Tri	BR	P	A	PL($\uparrow$/$\downarrow$)	Abd	Cre	Bab
R									
L									

0 = absent, 1+ = hypoactive, 2+ = normal, 3+ = hyperactive,
4+ = hyperactive with clonus, $\uparrow$ dorsiflexion, $\downarrow$ plantar flexion.

REGIONAL WRITE-UP—NEUROLOGICAL SYSTEM

Summarize your findings using the SOAP format.

Subjective (Reason for seeking care, health history)

Objective (Physical examination findings)   Record reflexes on diagram below

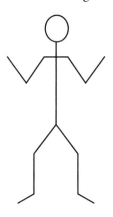

Assessment (Assessment of health state or problem, diagnosis)

Plan (Diagnostic evaluation, follow-up care, patient teaching)

NOTES

Chapter Twenty-Four

Male Genitourinary System

PURPOSE

This chapter helps you to learn the structure and function of the male genitalia; to learn the methods of inspection and palpation of these structures; and to record the assessment accurately.

READING ASSIGNMENT

Jarvis, *Physical Examination and Health Assessment*, 1st Canadian ed., Chapter 24, pp. 711–738.

AUDIO-VISUAL ASSIGNMENT

Jarvis, *Physical Examination and Health Assessment DVD Series: Male Genitalia*

GLOSSARY

Study the following terms after completing the reading assignment. You should be able to cover the definition on the right and define the term out loud.

Chancre ....red, round, superficial ulcer with a yellowish serous discharge that is a sign of syphilis

Condylomata acuminata ....soft, pointed, fleshy papules that occur on the genitalia and are caused by the human papillomavirus (HPV)

Cryptorchidism ....undescended testes

Cystitis ....inflammation of the urinary bladder

Epididymis ....structure composed of coiled ducts located over the superior and posterior surface of the testes, which stores sperm

Epispadias ....congenital defect in which urethra opens on the dorsal (upper) side of penis instead of at the tip

Hernia ....weak spot in abdominal muscle wall (usually in area of inguinal canal or femoral canal) through which a loop of bowel may protrude

Herpes genitalis...........................a sexually transmitted disease characterized by clusters of small painful vesicles, caused by a virus

Hydrocele ....cystic fluid in tunica vaginalis surrounding testis

Hypospadias ....congenital defect in which urethra opens on the ventral (under) side of penis rather than at the tip

Orchitis.......................................acute inflammation of testis, usually associated with mumps

Paraphimosis..............................foreskin is retracted and fixed behind the glans penis

Peyronie's disease......................nontender, hard plaques on the surface of penis, associated with painful bending of penis during erection

Phimosis....................................foreskin is advanced and tightly fixed over the glans penis

Prepuce......................................(foreskin) the hood or flap of skin over the glans penis that often is surgically removed after birth by circumcision

Priapism....................................prolonged, painful erection of penis without sexual desire

Spermatic cord ....collection of vas deferens, blood vessels, lymphatics, and nerves that ascends along the testis and through the inguinal canal into the abdomen

Spermatocele ....retention cyst in epididymis filled with milky fluid that contains sperm

Torsion.......................................sudden twisting of spermatic cord; a surgical emergency

Varicocele...................................dilated tortuous varicose veins in the spermatic cord

Vas deferens ....duct carrying sperm from the epididymis through the abdomen and then into the urethra

STUDY GUIDE

After completing the reading assignment and the audio-visual assignment, you should be able to answer the following questions in the space provided.

1. Describe the function of the cremaster muscle.

2. Identify the structures that provide transport of sperm.

3. Describe the significance of the inguinal canal and the femoral canal.

4. List the pros and cons of circumcision of the male newborn.

5. Discuss ways of creating an environment that will provide psychological comfort for the man and the examiner during examination of male genitalia.

6. List teaching points to include with the teaching of testicular self-examination.

7. Discuss the rationale for making certain that testes have descended in the male infant.

8. Contrast the physical appearance and clinical significance of these scrotal lumps:

   Epididymitis

   Varicocele

   Spermatocele

   Testicular tumour

   Hydrocele

9. Contrast the anatomical course and the clinical significance of these hernias:

Indirect inguinal

Direct inguinal

Femoral

Fill in the labels indicated on the following illustrations.

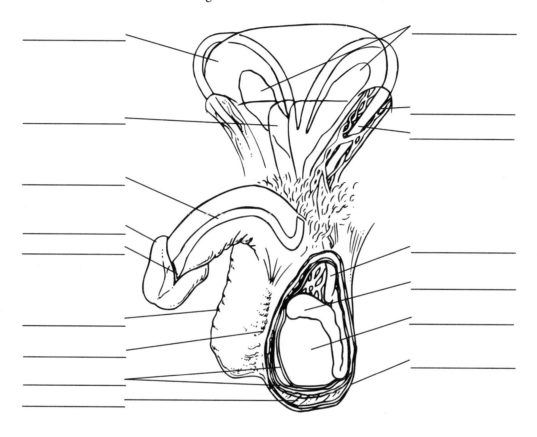

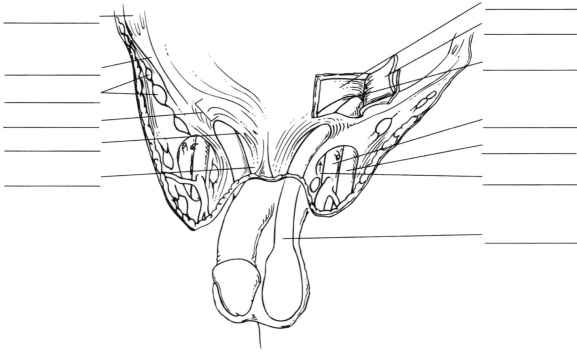

STRUCTURES OF THE INGUINAL AREA

REVIEW QUESTIONS

This test is for you to check your own mastery of the content. Answers are provided in Appendix A.

1. The examiner is going to inspect and palpate for a hernia. During this examination the man is instructed to:

   a. hold his breath during palpation.
   b. cough after the examiner has gently inserted the examination finger into the rectum.
   c. bear down when the examiner's finger is at the inguinal canal.
   d. relax in a supine position while the examination finger is inserted into the canal.

2. During examination of the scrotum, a normal finding would be:

   a. The left testicle is firmer to palpation than the right.
   b. The left testicle is larger than the right.
   c. The left testicle hangs lower than the right.
   d. The left testicle is more tender to palpation than the right.

3. H.T. has come to the clinic for a follow-up visit. Six months ago, he was started on a new medication. The class of medication is most likely to cause impotence as a side effect; therefore, medication classes explored by the nurse are:

   a. antipyretics.
   b. bronchodilators.
   c. corticosteroids.
   d. antihypertensives.

4. Prostatic hypertrophy occurs frequently in older men. The symptoms that may indicate this problem are:

   a. polyuria and urgency.
   b. dysuria and oliguria.
   c. straining, loss of force, and sense of residual urine.
   d. foul-smelling urine and dysuria.

5. A 64-year-old man has come for a health examination. A normal, age-related change in the scrotum would be:

   a. testicular atrophy.
   b. testicular hypertrophy.
   c. pendulous scrotum.
   d. increase in scrotal rugae.

6. During palpation of the testes, the normal finding would be:

   a. firm to hard, and rough.
   b. nodular.
   c. 2 to 3 cm long by 2 cm wide and firm.
   d. firm, rubbery, and smooth.

7. A 20-year-old man has indicated that he does not perform testicular self-examination. One of the facts that should be shared with him is that testicular cancer, though rare, does occur most commonly in men aged:

   a. under 15.
   b. 15 to 49.
   c. 50 to 65.
   d. 65 and older.

8. During the examination of a full-term new-born male, a finding requiring investigation would be:

   a. absent testes.
   b. meatus centred at the tip of the penis.
   c. wrinkled scrotum.
   d. penis 2 to 3 cm in length.

9. During transillumination of a scrotum, you note a nontender mass that transilluminates with a red glow. This finding is suggestive of:

   a. scrotal hernia.
   b. scrotal edema.
   c. orchitis.
   d. hydrocele.

10. How sensitive to pressure are normal testes?

    a. somewhat
    b. not at all
    c. left is more sensitive than right
    d. only when inflammation is present

11. The congenital displacement of the urethral meatus to the inferior surface of the penis is:

    a. hypospadias.
    b. epispadias.
    c. hypoesthesia.
    d. hypophysis.

12. An adhesion of the prepuce to the head of the penis, making it impossible to retract, is:

    a. paraphimosis.
    b. phimosis.
    c. smegma.
    d. dyschezia.

13. The first physical sign associated with puberty in boys is:

    a. height spurt.
    b. penis lengthening.
    c. sperm production.
    d. pubic hair development.
    e. testes enlargement.

14. Write a narrative account of an assessment of male genitalia with healthy findings.

SKILLS LABORATORY/CLINICAL SETTING

You are now ready for the clinical component of the male genitalia examination. Because of the need to maintain personal privacy, it is likely you will not practise this examination on a classmate. You will likely practise with a teaching mannequin in the skills laboratory or with a male in the clinical setting. Before you proceed, discuss the feelings that may be experienced by the man and the examiner and methods to increase the comfort of both. Make sure you have discussed the steps of the examination with your instructor before examining a patient.

CLINICAL OBJECTIVES

1. Demonstrate knowledge of the signs and symptoms related to the male genitalia by obtaining a pertinent health history.

2. Inspect and palpate the penis and scrotum.

3. Palpate the inguinal region for hernia.

4. Teach testicular self-examination.

5. Record the history and physical examination findings accurately, reach an assessment of the health state, and develop a plan of care.

INSTRUCTIONS

Prepare the examination setting and gather your equipment. Wash your hands; wear gloves during the examination. Practise the steps of the examination on a male in the clinical setting, giving appropriate instructions as you proceed. Record your findings using the regional write-up sheet that follows. The front of the page is intended as a worksheet; the back of the page is intended for your narrative summary recording using the SOAP format.

Note the student performance checklist that follows the regional write-up sheet. It lists the essential behaviours you should display as an examiner, and it may be used by your clinical instructor to evaluate your clinical teaching of testicular self-examination.

NOTES

REGIONAL WRITE-UP—MALE GENITOURINARY SYSTEM

Date _____

Examiner _____

Patient _____ Age _____ Gender _____

Occupation _____

I. Health History

	No	Yes, explain
1. Any urinary **frequency, urgency,** or waking during the night to urinate?	_____	_____
2. Any **pain** or **burning** with urinating?	_____	_____
3. Any **trouble starting urine stream**?	_____	_____
4. Urine **colour cloudy** or **foul-smelling**?	_____	_____
Red-tinged or **bloody**?	_____	_____
5. Any **problem controlling your urine**?	_____	_____
6. Any **pain** or **sores** on penis?	_____	_____
7. Any **lump** in testicles or scrotum?	_____	_____
Do you perform testicular self-examination?	_____	_____
8. In relationship now involving intercourse?	_____	_____
Use a contraceptive? Which one?	_____	_____
9. Any contact with partner who has a sexually transmitted infection?	_____	_____

II. Physical Examination

A. Inspect and palpate penis
Skin condition _____
Glans _____
Urethral meatus _____
Shaft _____

B. Inspect and palpate the scrotum
Skin condition _____
Testes _____
Spermatic cord _____
Transillumination (if indicated) _____

C. Inspect and palpate for hernia
Inguinal canal _____
Femoral area _____

D. Palpate inguinal lymph nodes

E. Teach testicular self-examination

REGIONAL WRITE-UP—MALE GENITOURINARY SYSTEM

Summarize your findings using the SOAP format.

Subjective (Reason for seeking care, health history)

Objective (Physical examination findings)

Assessment (Assessment of health state or problem, diagnosis)

Plan (Diagnostic evaluation, follow-up care, patient teaching)

STUDENT COMPETENCY CHECKLIST

TEACHING TESTICULAR SELF-EXAMINATION (TSE)

	S	U	Comments
I. Cognitive 1. Explain: a. why testicles are examined			
b. who should perform TSE			
c. frequency of testicular examination			
2. Describe the technique			
II. Performance			
1. Explains to male need for TSE			
2. Instructs male on technique of TSE by:			
a. describing method of palpating testicles			
b. describing normal findings			
c. describing abnormal findings to look for			
3. Instructs male to report unusual findings promptly			

NOTES

Chapter Twenty-Five

Anus, Rectum, and Prostate

PURPOSE

This chapter helps you to learn the structure and function of the anus and rectum and the male prostate gland; the methods of inspection and palpation of these structures; and how to record the assessment accurately.

READING ASSIGNMENT

Jarvis, *Physical Examination and Health Assessment,* 1st Canadian ed., Chapter 25, pp. 739–754.

AUDIO-VISUAL ASSIGNMENT

Jarvis, Physical Examination and Health Assessment DVD Series: Male Genitalia

GLOSSARY

Study the following terms after completing the reading assignment. You should be able to cover the definition on the right and define the term out loud.

Constipation...............................decrease in frequency of bowel movements, with difficult passing of very hard, dry stools

Fissure ....painful longitudinal tear in tissue, e.g., in the superficial mucosa at the anal margin

Hemorrhoid...............................flabby papules of skin or mucous membrane in the anal region caused by a varicose vein of the hemorrhoidal plexus

Melena ....blood in the stool

Pruritus......................................itching or burning sensation in the skin

Steatorrhea ....excessive fat in the stool as in gastrointestinal malabsorption of fat

Valves of Houston......................one of three semilunar transverse folds that cross one-half the circumference of the rectal lumen

STUDY GUIDE

After completing the reading assignment and the audio-visual assignment, you should be able to answer the following questions in the spaces provided.

1. State the length of the anal canal and the rectum in the adult, and describe the location of these structures in the lower abdomen.

2. Describe the size, shape, and location of the male prostate gland.

3. List a few examples of high-fibre foods of the soluble type and of the insoluble type; what advantages do these foods have for the body?

4. List screening measures that are recommended for early detection of colon or rectal cancer, and of prostate cancer.

5. State the method of promoting anal sphincter relaxation in order to aid palpation of the anus and rectum.

6. Describe the normal physical characteristics of the prostate gland that would be assessed by palpation:

Size

Shape

Surface

Consistency

Mobility

Sensitivity

7. Describe the physical appearance and clinical significance of a pilonidal cyst and an anorectal fistula.

8. Define the condition *benign prostatic hypertrophy*, list the usual symptoms the man experiences with this condition, and describe the physical characteristics.

Fill in the labels indicated on the following illustrations.

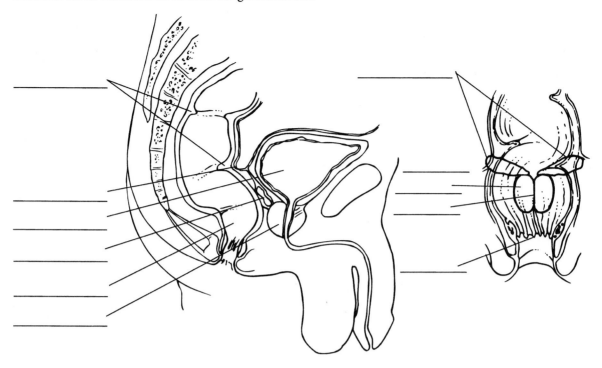

REVIEW QUESTIONS

This test is for you to check your own mastery of the content. Answers are provided in Appendix A.

1. The gastrocolic reflex is:

   a. a peristaltic wave.
   b. the passage of meconium in the newborn.
   c. another term for borborygmi.
   d. reverse peristalsis.

2. The incidence of benign prostatic hypertrophy (BPH):

   a. is highest among males aged 40 to 60 years.
   b. increases with age.
   c. decreases with age.
   d. is not related to age.

3. Select the best description of the anal canal.

   a. a 12-cm-long portion of the large intestine
   b. under involuntary control of the parasympathetic nervous system
   c. a 3.8-cm-long outlet of the gastrointestinal tract
   d. an S-shaped portion of the colon

4. While good nutrition is important for everyone, foods believed to help reduce risk of colon cancer are:

   a. high in fibre.
   b. low in fat.
   c. high in protein.
   d. high in carbohydrate.

5. Which finding in the prostate gland suggests prostate cancer?

    a. symmetrical smooth enlargement
    b. extreme tenderness to palpation
    c. boggy soft enlargement
    d. diffuse hardness

6. The bulbourethral gland is assessed:

    a. during an examination of a female patient.
    b. during an examination of both male and female patients.
    c. during an examination of a male patient.
    d. cannot be assessed with a rectal examination.

7. Inspection of stool is an important part of the rectal examination. Normal stool is:

    a. black in colour and tarry in consistency.
    b. brown in colour and soft in consistency.
    c. clay coloured and dry in consistency.
    d. varies depending upon the individual's diet.

8. Which symptoms suggest benign prostatic hypertrophy?

    a. weight loss and bone pain
    b. fever, chills, urinary frequency, and urgency
    c. difficulty initiating urination and weak stream
    d. dark, tarry stools

9. A false positive may occur on fecal occult blood tests of the stool if the person has ingested significant amounts of:

    a. red meat
    b. candies with red dye #2
    c. cranberry juice
    d. red beets

10. Write a narrative account of a rectal assessment with normal findings.

SKILLS LABORATORY/CLINICAL SETTING

You are now ready for the clinical component of the rectal examination. This regional examination usually is combined with the examination of the male genitalia or with examination of the female genitalia.

CLINICAL OBJECTIVES

1. Demonstrate knowledge of the signs and symptoms related to the rectal area by obtaining a pertinent health history.

2. Inspect and palpate the perianal region.

3. Test any stool specimen for occult blood.

4. Record the history and physical examination findings accurately.

INSTRUCTIONS

Prepare the examination setting and gather your equipment. Wash your hands; wear gloves during the examination; wash hands again after removing gloves. Practise the steps of the examination on a patient in the clinical setting, giving appropriate instructions as you proceed. Record your findings using the regional write-up sheet that follows. Note that only the worksheet is included in this chapter. Your narrative summary recording using the SOAP format can be included with the narrative summary of the genitalia.

NOTES

REGIONAL WRITE-UP—ANUS, RECTUM, AND PROSTATE GLAND

Date _____

Examiner _____

Patient _____ Age _____ Gender _____

Occupation _____

I. Health History

	No	Yes, explain
1. Bowels move **regularly**? How often?		
Usual colour? Hard or soft?		
2. Any **change** in usual bowel habits?		
3. Ever had **black or bloody stool**?		
4. Take any medications?		
5. Any **rectal itching, pain, or hemorrhoids**?		
6. Any family history of **colon/rectal polyps or cancer**?		
7. Describe usual amount of high-fibre foods in diet.		

II. Physical Examination

A. Inspect the perianal area
Skin condition _____
Sacrococcygeal area _____
Note skin integrity while patient performs Valsalva manoeuvre _____

B. Palpate anus and rectum
Anal sphincter _____
Anal canal _____
Rectal wall _____
Prostate gland (for males)
    Size _____
    Shape _____
    Surface _____
    Consistency _____
    Mobility _____
    Any tenderness _____
Cervix (for females) _____

C. Examination of stool
Visual inspection _____
Test for occult blood _____

NOTES

Female Genitourinary System

PURPOSE

This chapter helps you to learn the structure and function of the female genitalia; the methods of inspection and palpation of the internal and external structures; the procedures for collection of cytologic specimens; and to record the assessment accurately.

READING ASSIGNMENT

Jarvis, *Physical Examination and Health Assessment,* 1st Canadian ed., Chapter 26, pp. 755–792.

AUDIO-VISUAL ASSIGNMENT

Jarvis, *Physical Examination and Health Assessment DVD Series: Female Genitalia*

GLOSSARY

Study the following terms after completing the reading assignment. You should be able to cover the definition on the right and define the term out loud.

Adnexa..accessory organs of the uterus, that is, ovaries and fallopian tubes

Amenorrhea...............................absence of menstruation; termed secondary amenorrhea when menstruation has begun and then ceases; most common cause is pregnancy

Bartholin's glands ....vestibular glands, located on either side of the vaginal orifice, that secrete a clear lubricating mucus during intercourse

Bloody show...............................dislodging of thick cervical mucus plug at end of pregnancy, which is a sign of beginning of labour

Caruncle ....small, deep red mass protruding from urethral meatus, usually due to urethritis

Chadwick's sign ....bluish discoloration of cervix that occurs normally in pregnancy at six to eight weeks' gestation

Chancre ....red, round, superficial ulcer with a yellowish serous discharge that is a sign of syphilis

Clitoris...small, elongated, erectile tissue in the female, located at anterior juncture of labia minora

Cystocele.....................................prolapse of urinary bladder and its vaginal mucosa into the vagina with straining or standing

Dysmenorrhea............................abdominal cramping and pain associated with menstruation

Dyspareunia...............................painful intercourse

Dysuria ....painful urination

Endometriosis ....aberrant growths of endometrial tissue scattered throughout the pelvis

Fibroid..(myoma) hard painless nodules in uterine wall that cause uterine enlargement

Gonorrhea ....sexually transmitted infection characterized by purulent vaginal discharge, or may have no symptoms

Hegar's sign................................softening of cervix that is a sign of pregnancy, occurring at 10 to 12 weeks' gestation

Hematuria...................................red-tinged or bloody urine

Hymen ....membranous fold of tissue partly closing vaginal orifice

Leukorrhea ....whitish or yellowish discharge from vaginal orifice

Menarche ....onset of first menstruation, usually between 11 and 13 years of age

Menopause..................................cessation of the menses, usually occurring around 48 to 51 years

Menorrhagia...............................excessively heavy menstrual flow

Multipara ....condition of having two or more pregnancies

Nullipara ....condition of first pregnancy

Papanicolaou test ....painless test used to detect cervical cancer

Polyp...cervical polyp is bright red, soft, pedunculated growth emerging from os

Rectouterine pouch ....(cul-de-sac of Douglas) deep recess formed by the peritoneum between the rectum and cervix

Rectocele ....prolapse of rectum and its vaginal mucosa into vagina with straining or standing

Salpingitis ....inflammation of fallopian tubes

Skene's glands............................paraurethral glands

Vaginitis ....inflammation of vagina

Vulva ....external genitalia of female

STUDY GUIDE

After completing the reading assignment and the audio-visual assignment, you should be able to answer the following questions in the spaces provided.

1. List the external structures of the female genitalia.

2. Describe the size, shape, and location of the internal structures of the female genitalia.

3. Outline the changes observed during the perimenopausal period.

4. Discuss ways of creating an environment that will provide psychological comfort for both the woman and practitioner during the female genitalia examination.

5. Discuss selection, preparation, and insertion of the vaginal speculum.

6. Describe the appearance or sketch these normal variations of the cervix and os:

Nulliparous _____

Parous _____

Stellate lacerations _____

Cervical eversion _____

Nabothian cysts _____

7. List the steps in obtaining these specimens:

Cervical scrape using spatula

Endocervical specimen using cytobrush

8. When applying acetic acid (white vinegar) to the cervix and vaginal mucosa, list the normal response and the response suggesting infection.

9. Discuss the procedure and rationale for bimanual examination and list normal findings for the cervix, uterus, and adnexa.

10. Discuss infection control precautions during examination of female genitalia and procuring of specimens.

11. Describe or sketch the appearance of the following abnormalities of the cervix:

Chadwick's sign

Erosion

Polyp

Carcinoma

12. List the characteristics of vaginal discharge associated with the following conditions of vaginitis:

Atrophic vaginitis

Candidiasis

Trichomoniasis

Bacterial vaginosis

Chlamydia

Gonorrhea

13. Differentiate the signs and symptoms of these conditions of adnexal enlargement:

Ectopic pregnancy

Ovarian cyst

Fill in the labels indicated on the following illustrations.

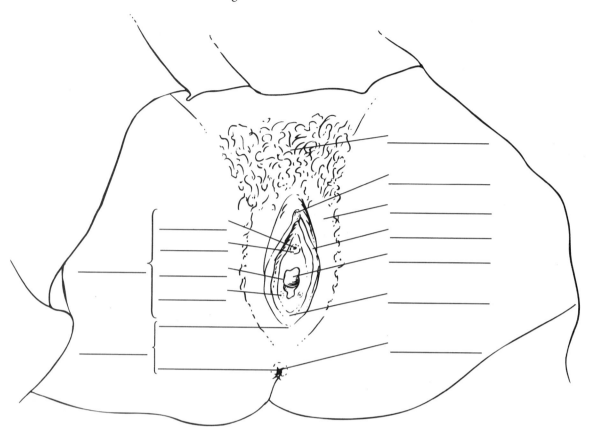

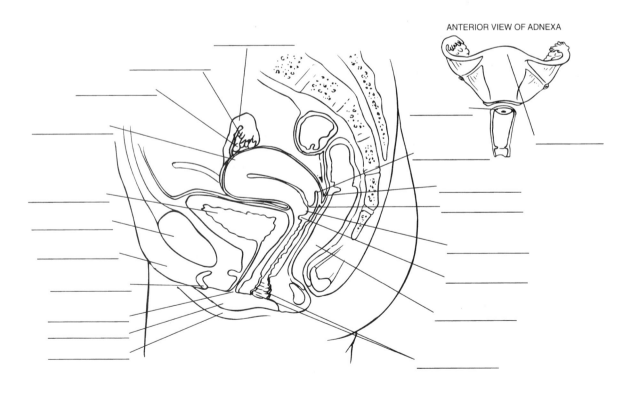

ANTERIOR VIEW OF ADNEXA

REVIEW QUESTIONS

This test is for you to check your own mastery of the content. Answers are provided in Appendix A.

1. Vaginal lubrication is provided during intercourse by:

   a. the labia minora.
   b. sebaceous follicles.
   c. Skene's glands.
   d. Bartholin's glands.

2. A young woman has come for her first gynecological examination. Because the patient has not had any children, the examiner would expect the cervical os to appear:

   a. smooth and circular.
   b. irregular and slit-like.
   c. irregular and circular.
   d. smooth and enlarged.

3. A woman has come for an examination because of a missed menstrual period and a positive home pregnancy test. Examination reveals a cervix that appears cyanotic. This is referred to as:

   a. Goodell's sign.
   b. Hegar's sign.
   c. Tanner's sign.
   d. Chadwick's sign.

4. During the examination of the genitalia of a 70-year-old woman, a normal finding would be:

   a. hypertrophy of the mons pubis.
   b. increase in vaginal secretions.
   c. thin and sparse pubic hair.
   d. bladder prolapse.

5. For a woman, history of her mother's health during pregnancy is important. A medication that requires frequent follow-up is:

   a. corticosteroid.
   b. theophylline.
   c. diethylstilbestrol.
   d. aminoglycoside.

6. A woman has come for health care complaining of a thick, white discharge with intense itching. These symptoms are suggestive of:

   a. atrophic vaginitis.
   b. trichomoniasis.
   c. chlamydia.
   d. candidiasis.

7. To prepare the vaginal speculum for insertion, the examiner:

   a. lubricates it with a water-soluble lubricant.
   b. lubricates it with petrolatum.
   c. warms it under the light, then inserts it into the vagina.
   d. lubricates it with warm water.

8. To insert the speculum as comfortably as possible, the examiner:

   a. opens the speculum slightly and inserts in an upward direction.
   b. presses the introitus down with one hand and inserts the blades obliquely with the other.
   c. spreads the labia with one hand, inserts the closed speculum horizontally with the other.
   d. pushes down on the introitus and inserts the speculum in an upward direction.

9. Before withdrawing the speculum, the examiner swabs the cervix with a swab soaked in acetic acid. This examination is done to assess for:

   a. herpes simplex virus.
   b. contact dermatitis.
   c. human papillomavirus.
   d. carcinoma.

10. Select the best description of the uterus.

   a. anteverted, round asymmetrical organ
   b. pear-shaped, thick-walled organ flattened anteroposteriorly
   c. retroverted, almond-shaped asymmetrical organ
   d. midposition, thick-walled oval organ

11. In placing a finger on either side of the cervix and moving it side to side, you are assessing:

   a. the diameter of the fallopian tube.
   b. cervical motion tenderness.
   c. the ovaries.
   d. the uterus.

12. Which of the following is (are) normal, common finding(s) on inspection and palpation of the vulva and perineum?

   a. labia majora that are wide apart and gaping
   b. palpable Bartholin's glands
   c. clear, thin discharge from paraurethral glands
   d. bulging at introitus during Valsalva manoeuvre

13. Which of the following is the most common bacterial sexually transmitted infection in Canada?

   a. human papillomavirus
   b. gonorrhea
   c. trichomoniasis
   d. syphilis
   e. bacterial vaginosis

14. Write a narrative account of an assessment of female genitalia with normal findings.

SKILLS LABORATORY/CLINICAL SETTING

You are now ready for the clinical component of the female genitalia examination. Because of the need to maintain personal privacy, it is likely you will not practise this examination on a peer. Your practice likely will be with a teaching mannequin in the skills laboratory or with a woman in the clinical setting under the guidance of a preceptor. Before you proceed, discuss the feelings that may be experienced by the woman and examiner and methods to increase the comfort of both. With your instructor, discuss methods of positioning the woman, steps in using the vaginal speculum, steps in procuring specimens, and methods of infection control precautions.

CLINICAL OBJECTIVES

1. Demonstrate knowledge of the signs and symptoms related to the female genitalia by obtaining a pertinent health history.

2. Demonstrate measures to increase the woman's comfort before and during the examination.

3. Demonstrate knowledge of infection control precautions before, during, and after the examination.

4. Inspect and palpate the external genitalia.

5. Using the vaginal speculum, gather materials for cytological study.

6. Inspect and palpate the internal genitalia.

7. Record the history and physical examination findings accurately, reach an assessment of the health state, and develop a plan of care.

INSTRUCTIONS

Prepare the examination setting and gather your equipment. Collect the health history before the woman disrobes for the examination. Wash your hands; wear gloves during the examination; wash hands again after removing gloves. Practise the steps of the examination on a woman in the clinical setting, giving appropriate instructions as you proceed. Record your findings using the regional write-up sheet that follows. The first section is intended as a worksheet; the last page is intended for your narrative summary recording using the SOAP format. Collection of data for the rectal examination is usually combined with the examination of female genitalia; see Chapter 25 for the regional write-up sheet for the rectal examination.

NOTES

REGIONAL WRITE-UP—FEMALE GENITOURINARY SYSTEM

Date _____

Examiner _____

Patient _____ Age _____ Gender _____

Occupation _____

I. Health History

	No	Yes, explain
1. Date of **last menstrual period?**		
Age at first period? Usual cycle?		
Duration? Usual amount of flow?		
Any pain or cramps with period?		
2. Ever been **pregnant**? How many times?		
Describe pregnancy(ies)		
Any complications?		
3. Periods slowed down or **stopped**?		
4. How often has **gynecological checkup**?		
Date of last Pap test? Results?		
5. Any problems with **urinating**?		
6. Any unusual **vaginal discharge**?		
7. **Sores** or **lesions** in genitals?		
8. In relationship now involving intercourse?		
9. Use a contraceptive? Which one?		
10. Any contact with partner who has a sexually transmitted infection?		
11. Any precautions to reduce risk of STIs?		
12. Taking any medications?		
Any hormone therapy?		

II. Physical Examination
A. Inspect external genitalia

Skin colour and characteristics _____

Hair distribution _____

Symmetry _____

Clitoris _____

Labia _____

Urethral opening _____

Vaginal opening _____

Perineum _____

Jarvis, Luctkar-Flude: PHYSICAL EXAMINATION AND HEALTH ASSESSMENT, First Canadian Edition, Student Laboratory Manual. Copyright © 2009 by Elsevier Canada, a division of Reed Elsevier Canada, Ltd. All rights reserved.

B. Palpate external genitalia

Skene's glands _____

Bartholin's glands _____

Perineum _____

Assess perineal muscle strength _____

Assess for vaginal wall bulging or urinary incontinence _____

Discharge and characteristics _____

C. Speculum examination

Inspect cervix and os

    Colour _____

    Position _____

    Size _____

    Surface _____

    Discharge and characteristics _____

Obtain cervical smears and cultures

    Vaginal pool _____

    Cervical scrape _____

    Endocervical specimen _____

    Other (if indicated) _____

Complete acetic acid wash _____

Inspect vaginal wall as speculum is removed _____

D. Bimanual examination

Cervix

    Consistency _____

    Mobility _____

    Tenderness with motion _____

Uterus

    Size and shape _____

    Consistency _____

    Position _____

    Mobility _____

    Tenderness _____

Adnexa _____

    Able to palpate? (Be honest.) _____

    Size and shape of ovaries _____

    Tenderness _____

    Masses _____

Rectovaginal examination _____

REGIONAL WRITE-UP—FEMALE GENITOURINARY SYSTEM

Summarize your findings using the SOAP format.

Subjective (Reason for seeking care, health history)

Objective (Physical examination findings)   Record findings on diagram below.

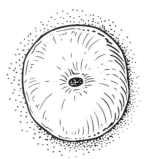

Assessment (Assessment of health state or problem, diagnosis)

Plan (Diagnostic evaluation, follow-up care, patient teaching)

NOTES

UNIT 4

Integration of the Health Assessment

27

The Complete Health Assessment: Putting It All Together

PURPOSE

This chapter helps you to learn the methods of integrating the regional examinations so that you will be able to conduct a complete physical examination on a well young adult.

READING ASSIGNMENT

Jarvis, *Physical Examination and Health Assessment,* 1st Canadian ed., Chapter 27, pp. 793–814.

_____

AUDIO-VISUAL ASSIGNMENT

Jarvis, Physical Examination and Health Assessment DVD Series: Head-to-Toe Examination of the Adult

_____

263

CLINICAL OBJECTIVES

1. Demonstrate skills of inspection, percussion, palpation, and auscultation.

2. Demonstrate correct use of instruments, including assembly, manipulation of component parts, and positioning with patient.

3. Use appropriate terminology and correctly pronounce medical terminology with clinical instructor and with patient.

4. Choreograph the complete examination in a systematic manner, including integration of certain regional assessments throughout the examination (for example: skin, musculoskeletal).

5. Coordinate procedures to limit position changes for examiner and patient.

6. Describe accurately the findings of the examination, including normal and abnormal findings.

7. Demonstrate appropriate infection control measures.

8. Recognize and maintain the privacy and dignity of the patient.
   a. Adequately explain what is being done while limiting small talk.
   b. Consider patient's anxiety and fears.
   c. Consider your own facial expression and comments.
   d. Demonstrate confidence, empathy, and gentle manner.
   e. Acknowledge and apologize for any discomfort caused.
   f. Provide for privacy and warmth at all times.
   g. Determine comfort level, pausing if patient becomes tired.
   h. Wash hands and don gloves appropriately.
   i. Allow adequate time for each step.
   j. Briefly summarize findings to patient, and thank patient for his or her time.

INSTRUCTIONS

The key to success in this venture is practice; you should conduct at least three complete physical examination practices in your preparation for this final examination proficiency. You are responsible for obtaining a peer "patient" for the examination. You should prepare your own note card "outline" for the examination. You may refer to this minimally during the examination, but overdependence on your notes will constitute failure. You will have 45 minutes in which to conduct the examination (not including setup). Genitalia examination is omitted. If you practise three times, you will have no difficulty completing the examination in the alloted time.

Prepare the examination setting. Arrange for proper lighting. If you are using a hospital bed instead of an examination table, make sure to adjust the bed height during the examination to allow for your own visualization of the patient, and for the patient's ease in getting into and out of the bed. Arrange adequate patient gown, bath blankets, and drapes.

Gather your equipment. The following items are needed for a complete physical examination, including female genitalia. Check with your clinical instructor for any items that you may omit for your own examination proficiency.

Platform scale with height attachment
Sphygmomanometer with appropriate size cuff
Stethoscope with bell and diaphragm endpieces
Alcohol wipes for cleaning equipment
Thermometer
Flashlight or penlight
Otoscope/ophthalmoscope
Tuning fork
Nasal speculum
Tongue depressor
Pocket vision screener
Skin-marking pen
Flexible tape measure and ruler marked in centimetres
Reflex hammer
Sharp object (split tongue blade)
Cotton balls
Bivalve vaginal speculum
Disposable gloves
Materials for cytological study
Lubricant
Fecal occult blood test materials

Record your findings using the write-up sheets that follow. Your clinical instructor may ask you to record your findings ahead of time, following one of your practice sessions. Then you can give your write-up to the instructor to follow along as you perform the final examination proficiency.

Good luck!

NOTES

COMPLETE PHYSICAL EXAMINATION

Date _____

Examiner _____

Patient _____ Age _____ Gender _____

Occupation _____

General Survey of Patient

1. Appears stated age _____
2. Level of consciousness _____
3. Skin colour _____
4. Nutritional status _____
5. Posture and position _____
6. Obvious physical deformities _____
7. Mobility: gait, use of assistive devices, ROM of joints, no involuntary movement _____
8. Facial expression _____
9. Mood and affect _____
10. Speech: articulation, pattern, content appropriate, native language _____
11. Hearing _____
12. Personal hygiene _____

Measurement and Vital Signs

1. Weight _____
2. Height _____
3. Body mass index _____
4. Vision using Snellen eye chart _____
   Right eye _____ Left eye _____ Correction? _____
5. Radial pulse, rate, and rhythm _____
6. Respirations, rate, depth _____
7. Blood pressure
   Right arm _____ (sitting or lying?)
   Left arm _____ (sitting or lying?)
8. Temperature (if indicated) _____
9. Pain assessment _____

STAND IN FRONT OF PATIENT, PATIENT IS SITTING

Skin

1. Hands and nails _____
2. (For remainder of examination, examine skin with corresponding region)
   Colour and pigmentation _____
   Temperature _____
   Moisture _____
   Texture _____
   Turgor _____
   Any lesions _____

Head and Face

1. Scalp, hair, cranium _____
2. Face (cranial nerve VII) _____
3. Temporal artery, temporomandibular joint _____
4. Maxillary sinuses, frontal sinuses _____

Eyes

1. Visual fields (cranial nerve II) _____
2. Extraocular muscles, corneal light reflex _____
   Cardinal positions of gaze (cranial nerves III, IV, VI) _____
3. External structures _____
4. Conjunctivae _____
   Sclerae _____
   Corneas _____
   Irides _____
5. Pupils _____
6. Ophthalmoscope, red reflex _____
   Disc _____
   Vessels _____
   Retinal background _____

Ears

1. External ear _____
2. Any tenderness _____
3. Otoscope, ear canal _____
   Tympanic membrane _____
4. Test hearing (cranial nerve VIII), voice test _____
   Weber test _____
   Rinne test _____

Nose

1. External nose _____
2. Patency of nostrils _____
3. Speculum, nasal mucosa _____
   Septum _____
   Turbinates _____

Mouth and Throat

1. Lips and buccal mucosa _____
   Teeth and gums _____
   Tongue _____
   Hard/soft palate _____
2. Tonsils _____
3. Uvula (cranial nerves IX, X) _____
4. Tongue (cranial nerve XII) _____

Neck
1. Symmetry, lumps, pulsations _____
2. Cervical lymph nodes _____
3. Carotid pulse (bruits if indicated) _____
4. Trachea _____
5. ROM and muscle strength (cranial nerve XI) _____

MOVE TO BACK OF PATIENT, PATIENT SITTING

6. Thyroid gland _____

Chest and Lungs, Posterior and Lateral
1. Thoracic cage configuration _____
   Skin characteristics _____
   Symmetry _____
2. Symmetric expansion _____
   Tactile fremitus _____
   Lumps or tenderness _____
3. Spinous processes _____
4. Percussion over lung fields _____
   Diaphragmatic excursion _____
5. CVA tenderness _____
6. Breath sounds _____
7. Adventitious sounds _____

MOVE TO FRONT OF PATIENT

Chest and Lungs, Anterior
1. Respirations and skin characteristics _____
2. Tactile fremitus, lumps, tenderness _____
3. Percuss lung fields _____
4. Breath sounds _____

Upper Extremities
1. ROM and muscle strength _____
2. Epitrochlear nodes _____

Breasts
1. Symmetry, mobility, dimpling _____
2. Supraclavicular and infraclavicular areas _____

PATIENT SUPINE, STAND AT PATIENT'S RIGHT

3. Breast palpation _____
4. Nipple _____
5. Axillae and regional nodes _____
6. Teach breast self-examination _____

Neck Vessels
1. Jugular venous pulse _____
2. Jugular venous pressure, if indicated _____

Heart
1. Precordium: pulsations and heave _____
2. Apical impulse _____
3. Precordium, thrills _____
4. Apical rate and rhythm _____
5. Heart sounds _____

Abdomen
1. Contour, symmetry _____
   Skin characteristics _____
   Umbilicus and pulsations _____
2. Bowel sounds _____
3. Vascular sounds _____
4. Percussion _____
5. Liver span in right MCL _____
6. Spleen _____
7. Light and deep palpation _____
8. Palpation of liver, spleen, kidneys, aorta _____
9. Abdominal reflexes, if indicated _____

Inguinal Area
1. Femoral pulse _____
2. Inguinal nodes _____

Lower Extremities
1. Symmetry _____
   Skin characteristics, hair distribution _____
2. Pulses, popliteal _____
   Posterior tibial _____
   Dorsalis pedis _____
3. Temperature, pretibial edema _____
4. Toes _____

PATIENT SITS UP
5. ROM and muscle strength, hips _____
   Knees _____
   Ankles and feet _____

Neurological
1. Sensation, face _____
   Arms and hands _____
   Legs and feet _____
2. Position sense _____
3. Stereognosis _____
4. Cerebellar function, finger-to-nose _____
5. Cerebellar function, heel-to-shin _____
6. Deep tendon reflexes
   Biceps _____   Triceps _____

Brachioradialis _____   Patellar _____

Achilles _____

7. Babinski reflex _____

PATIENT STANDS UP

Musculoskeletal

1. Walk across room _____

Walk, heel to toe _____

2. Walk on tiptoes, then walk on heels _____

3. Romberg sign _____

4. Shallow knee bend _____

5. Touch toes _____

6. ROM of spine _____

Male Genitalia

1. Penis and scrotum _____

2. Testes and spermatic cord _____

3. Inguinal hernia _____

4. Teach testicular self-examination _____

Male Rectum

1. Perianal area _____

2. Rectal walls and prostate gland _____

3. Stool for occult blood _____

FEMALE PATIENT IN LITHOTOMY POSITION

Female Genitalia and Rectum

1. Perineal and perianal areas _____

2. Vaginal speculum: cervix and vaginal walls _____

3. Procure specimens _____

4. Bimanual: cervix, uterus, and adnexa _____

_____

5. Rectovaginal _____

6. Stool for occult blood _____

Closure

1. Help patient sit up

2. Thank patient for time and depart from patient

NOTES

Chapter Twenty-Eight

Reassessment of the Hospitalized Adult

PURPOSE

This chapter helps you to learn the methods of integrating the regional examinations in the manner that suits the inpatient setting. The selection and sequencing of the techniques included are structured to provide an assessment that is efficient, thorough, and consistent with the assessments performed by other nurses in the course of 24-hour care.

READING ASSIGNMENT

Jarvis, *Physical Examination and Health Assessment,* 1st Canadian ed., Chapter 28, pp. 815–819.

CLINICAL OBJECTIVES

1. Demonstrate skills of inspection, percussion, palpation, and auscultation.

2. Demonstrate correct use of instruments, including assembly, manipulation of component parts, and positioning with patient.

3. Use appropriate terminology and correctly pronounce medical terminology with clinical instructor and with patient.

4. Choreograph the complete examination in a systematic manner, including integration of certain regional assessments throughout the examination (for example: skin, musculoskeletal).

5. Coordinate procedures to limit position changes for examiner and patient.

6. Describe accurately the findings of the examination, including normal and abnormal findings.

7. Demonstrate appropriate infection control measures.

8. Recognize and maintain the privacy and dignity of the patient.

  a. Adequately explain what is being done while limiting small talk.
  b. Consider patient's anxiety and fears.
  c. Consider your own facial expression and comments.
  d. Demonstrate confidence, empathy, and gentle manner.
  e. Acknowledge and apologize for any discomfort caused.
  f. Provide for privacy and warmth at all times.
  g. Determine comfort level, pausing if patient becomes tired.
  h. Wash hands and don gloves appropriately.
  i. Allow adequate time for each step.
  j. Briefly summarize findings to patient, and thank patient for his or her time.

9. Complete all procedures with attention to specifics of technique, which allows clear and consistent replication of the procedures by others assessing the same patient.

INSTRUCTIONS

As with other assessments, this particular version of the head-to-toe examination requires a great deal of practice before you will feel truly confident. The good news about this sequence is that it is directly applicable in any inpatient clinical sites that you attend, which is likely to be most of them. If you are already attending clinicals, use any available time to practise this sequence on real patients.

You are responsible for recruiting a friend or classmate to act as your patient for this examination. Prepare an outline on a note card to help you remember the sequence. Don't use it as a step-by-step instruction, but rather as a double-check so that you do not omit anything. Once this examination is over, you can take the note card with you to clinicals and use it as a reference.

You will have 20 minutes for this examination, not including setup. If you have practised the individual regional assessments thoroughly and can complete this particular sequence three times, you will be able to complete it satisfactorily within the time allotted.

Prepare the examination setting. Arrange the lighting, furniture, and bed to allow for the most efficient and comfortable activity for yourself and your patient. Think carefully about the functions of the patient's hospital bed. It can be useful to raise the bed closer to your eyes and stethoscope, but you cannot expect the patient to get out of bed safely from that height. Position sheets, drapes, and bath blankets strategically to achieve the proper balance of modesty, efficiency, and comfort.

Gather and arrange your equipment before you begin. The following items are needed for this sequence, but your instructor may modify the equipment list slightly for your individual class or exercise.

Water (in a cup)
Watch with a second hand
Stethoscope
Blood pressure cuff
Pulse oximeter
Penlight
Ruler in millimetres

Oxygen equipment (as indicated by your instructor)
Doppler (as indicated by your instructor)
Bladder scanner (as indicated by your instructor)
Standardized scales to calculate patient's risk for skin breakdown and falling
Documentation forms (as included here, or provided by your instructor)

Verify with your instructor whether you should submit documentation of this particular assessment after your demonstration or documentation that you have prepared to reflect one of your earlier practice sessions.

Good luck!

NOTES

COMPLETE INPATIENT REASSESSMENT

Date _____

Examiner _____

Patient _____ Age _____ Gender _____

Occupation _____

Introduction
1. Check for flags or markers at doorway
2. Introduce yourself
3. Perform hand hygiene
4. Make eye contact
5. Offer water
6. Check name band
7. Ask appropriate interview questions
8. Elevate the bed to appropriate height

General Appearance
1. Facial expression _____
2. Body position _____
3. Level of consciousness _____
4. Skin colour _____
5. Nutritional status _____
6. Speech: articulation, pattern, content appropriate _____
7. Hearing _____
8. Personal hygiene _____

Measurement
1. Temperature _____
2. Pulse _____
3. Respiration _____
4. Blood pressure _____
5. Pulse oximetry (oxygen saturation) _____
6. Weight on admission or if daily weight is indicated _____
7. Rate pain level on 0 to 10 scale; note ability to tolerate pain _____
8. Pain reassessment, if appropriate to scenario _____

Neurological System
1. Eyes open:
   a. Spontaneously _____
   b. Name _____
2. Motor response _____
3. Verbal response _____
4. Pupil size in mm and reaction
   a. R _____ b. L _____
5. Muscle strength, upper
   a. R _____ b. L _____

6. Muscle strength, lower
   a. R _____   b. L _____
7. Any ptosis, facial droop _____
8. Sensation _____
9. Communication _____
10. Ability to swallow _____

Respiratory

1. Oxygen by mask, nasal prongs; check fitting _____
2. FiO_2 _____
3. Respiratory effort _____
4. Auscultate breath sounds:
   Anterior lobes:
      Right upper _____
      Left upper _____
      Right middle _____
      Right lower _____
      Left lower _____
   Posterior lobes:
      Left upper _____
      Right upper _____
      Left lower _____
      Right lower _____
   Cough and deep breathe; any mucus? Check colour and amount _____

Cardiovascular System

1. Auscultate rhythm at apex: regular, irregular? _____
2. Check apical versus radial pulse
3. Assess heart sounds in all auscultatory areas: first with diaphragm, repeat with bell
4. Check capillary refill _____
5. Check pretibial edema
   a. R _____   b. L _____
6. Palpate posterior tibial pulse
   a. R _____   b. L _____
7. Palpate dorsalis pedis pulse
   a. R _____   b. L _____
8. Pulses by Doppler, if assigned _____
9. IV fluid and rate, if present _____

Skin (may be integrated with rest of assessment)

1. Colour _____
2. Temperature _____
3. Pinch up a fold of skin under the clavicle or on the forearm _____
4. Standardized scale regarding skin breakdown _____
5. Settings and application of specialized surface, if present _____

Abdomen

1. Contour of abdomen: flat, rounded, protuberant _____
2. Bowel sounds in all four quadrants _____
3. Check any tube drainage and site _____
4. Inquire if passing flatus or stool _____

Genitourinary
1. Inquire if voiding regularly _____
2. Urine for colour, clarity _____
3. Bladder scan, if indicated _____

Activity
1. Transfer to chair _____
2. Note any assistance needed, how movement is tolerated, distance walked to chair, ability to turn

   _____
3. Need for any ambulatory aid or equipment _____
4. Standardized scale regarding falling _____

Closure
1. Return bed to lowest height
2. Verify that brakes are locked
3. Make sure appropriate rails are up
4. Ensure call bell is available
5. Verify bed alarm, if indicated
6. Thank the patient for his or her attention and cooperation

NOTES

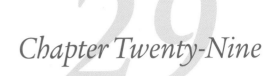

Chapter Twenty-Nine

Pregnancy

PURPOSE

This chapter helps you learn the changes and function of the female genitalia during pregnancy; the methods of inspection and palpation of the internal and external structures and the maternal abdomen; and how to record the assessment accurately.

READING ASSIGNMENT

Jarvis, *Physical Examination and Health Assessment,* 1st Canadian ed., Chapter 29, pp. 821–854.

AUDIO-VISUAL ASSIGNMENT

Jarvis, *Physical Examination and Health Assessment DVD Series: Head-to-Toe Examination of the Pregnant Woman*

GLOSSARY

Study the following terms after completing the reading assignment. You should be able to cover the definition on the right and define the term out loud.

Amniocentesis ....the transabdominal perforation of the amniotic sac for the purpose of obtaining a sample of amniotic fluid

Antepartum ....the period occurring before childbirth

Blastocyst ....the fertilized ovum; a specialized layer of cells around the blastocyst becomes the placenta

Chadwick's sign ....bluish/purple discoloration of the cervix during pregnancy due to venous congestion

Chloasma ....the "mask of pregnancy"; butterfly-shaped pigmentation of the face

Chorionic villi sampling ....transabdominal or transvaginal sampling of trophoblastic tissue surrounding the gestational sac

Colostrum ....the precursor to milk that contains minerals, proteins, and antibodies

Corpus luteum............................"yellow body": a structure on the surface of the ovary that is formed by the remaining cells in the follicle; it acts as a short-lived endocrine organ that produces progesterone to help maintain the pregnancy in its early stages

Diastasis recti ....separation of the abdominal muscles during pregnancy, returning to normal after pregnancy

Engagement ....when the widest diameter of the presenting part has descended into the pelvic inlet

Fetal lie ....orientation of the fetal spine to the maternal spine

Goodell's sign ....the softening of the cervix due to increased vascularity, congestion, and edema

Hegar's sign...............................when the uterus becomes globular in shape, softens, and flexes easily over the cervix

Hyperemesis gravidarum..........severe and debilitating nausea and vomiting that may persist beyond the 14th week of pregnancy and cause dehydration, weight loss, and electrolyte imbalance

Intrapartum...............................occurring during labour and delivery

Leopold's manoeuvre ....external palpation of the maternal abdomen to determine fetal lie, presentation, attitude, and position

Linea nigra ....a median line of the abdomen that becomes pigmented (darkens) during pregnancy

"Morning sickness" ....nausea and vomiting of pregnancy that usually begins between weeks 4 and 6, peaks between weeks 8 and 12, and resolves between weeks 14 and 16

Mucus plug................................mucus that forms a thick barrier in the cervix that is expelled at various times before or during labour

Multigravida..............................a pregnant woman who has previously carried a fetus to the point of viability

Multipara ....a woman who has had two or more viable pregnancies and deliveries

Nägele's rule..............................a rule for calculating the estimated date of delivery; add seven days to the first day of the last menstrual period and subtract three months

Pelvimetry.................................assessment of the maternal pelvis bones for shape and size

Pica ....a craving for unnatural articles of food, such as cornstarch and ice chips

Position ....the location of a fetal part to the right or left of the maternal pelvis

Postpartum...............................the period occurring after delivery

Presentation ....the part of the fetus that is entering the pelvis first

Primigravida ....a woman pregnant for the first time

Jarvis, Luctkar-Flude: PHYSICAL EXAMINATION AND HEALTH ASSESSMENT, First Canadian Edition, Student Laboratory Manual. Copyright © 2009 by Elsevier Canada, a division of Reed Elsevier Canada, Ltd. All rights reserved.

Primipara...................................a woman who has had one pregnancy and delivery

Striae gravidarum......................"stretch marks" that may be seen on the abdomen and breasts (in areas of weight gain) during pregnancy

VBAC ....vaginal birth after Caesarean delivery

STUDY GUIDE

After completing the reading assignment and the audio-visual assignment, you should be able to answer the following questions in the spaces provided.

1. Describe the function of the placenta.

2. Using Nägele's rule, calculate the estimated date of delivery if the LMP is August 22.

3. Give examples of the following signs of pregnancy.

   Presumptive:

   Probable:

   Positive:

4. When can serum hCG be detected in maternal blood?

5. Describe three physical and physiological changes that are seen in the:

   First trimester:

   Second trimester:

   Third trimester:

6. Describe the "expected" weight gain during pregnancy.

7. List the major concerns for teenage maternal morbidity and mortality.

8. List at least three risk factors concerning pregnant women of advanced maternal age.

9. Discuss the importance of ethnocultural differences and their role in a woman's pregnancy.

10. Discuss how using a relational approach to nursing allows you to provide culturally safe care to a woman during pregnancy.

11. True or False: Please circle the best answer.

    (1) True   False   A woman who has had a classical uterine incision is a good candidate for a VBAC.

    (2) True   False   In early fetal development, the corpus luteum plays no significance.

    (3) True   False   A woman who is pregnant for the first time is called a primipara.

    (4) True   False   The fetal period begins after the ninth gestational week.

    (5) True   False   Pre-eclampsia is seen only in the third trimester of pregnancy.

    (6) True   False   Vaginal bleeding in pregnancy always indicates a miscarriage.

    (7) True   False   Cervical incompetence is always accompanied by painful contractions.

12. What is the importance of fetal movement counting, and when should it be initiated?

13. Describe why it is important to ask a pregnant woman if she feels safe in her relationships and environment.

14. Draw on this diagram where the fundal height should be at the 20th week of gestation.

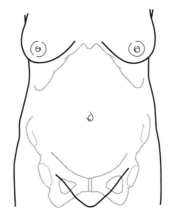

15. Label the following types of pelvis.

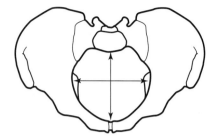

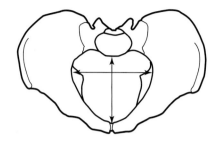

_____   _____

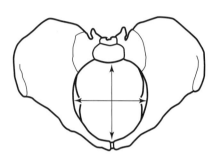

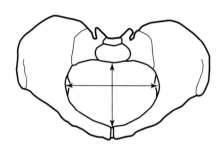

_____   _____

16. Label, list the order, and describe the purpose of the following _____ manoeuvres. (Fill in above blank.)

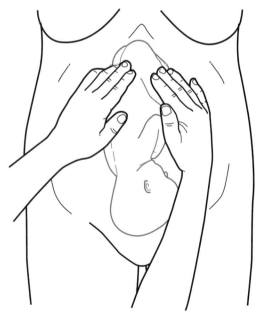

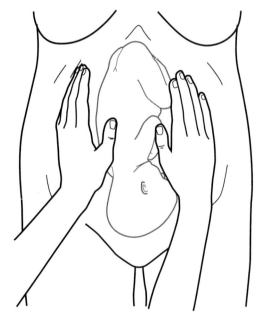

_____   _____

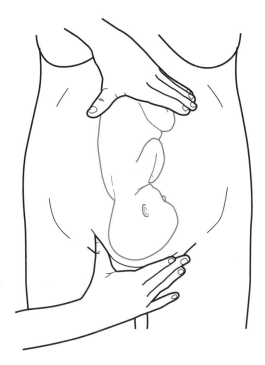

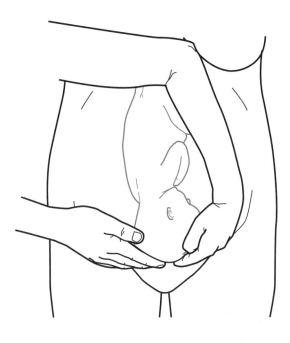

_____   _____

17. Describe the following for this figure.

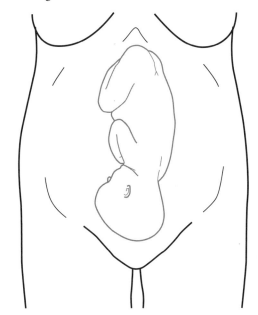

Fetal lie: _____

Fetal presentation: _____

Fetal position: _____

18. List the symptoms of pre-eclampsia.

19. List at least two reasons why fundal height may be small for gestational age.

20. List at least two reasons why fundal height may be large for gestational age.

REVIEW QUESTIONS

This test is for you to check your own mastery of the content. Answers are provided in Appendix A.

1. Ovulation begins on the:

   a. first day of the menstrual cycle.
   b. 28th day of the menstrual cycle.
   c. 14th day, approximately, of the menstrual cycle.

2. Using Nägele's rule, if a woman's last menstrual period started on January 13, the estimated date of delivery (EDD) is:

   a. $1/13 + 7 = 20$ $20 - 3$ months   EDD = October $\approx$ 29
   b. $1/13 + 10 = 23$ $23 - 3$ months   EDD = October $\approx$ 18
   c. $1/13 + 14 = 27$ $27 - 3$ months   EDD = September 30

3. A woman comes to the clinic complaining of nausea, fatigue, breast tenderness, urinary frequency, and amenorrhea. These are:

   a. probable signs of pregnancy.
   b. positive signs of pregnancy.
   c. presumptive signs of pregnancy.
   d. signs of stress.

4. After implantation, what structure makes progesterone to support the pregnancy up until week 10?

   a. corpus luteum
   b. blastocyst
   c. placenta
   d. ovary

5. Approximately two to three weeks before labour, the woman will experience:

   a. extreme fatigue.
   b. Braxton-Hicks contractions.
   c. lightening.
   d. back pain.

6. Cardiac output in a pregnant woman:

   a. drops dramatically.
   b. remains the same.
   c. increases along with stroke volume.
   d. decreases along with stroke volume.
   e. none of the above.

7. The pregnant adolescent is medically at risk for:

   a. poor weight gain, pre-eclampsia, thyroiditis, miscarriage.
   b. poor weight gain, pre-eclampsia, and sexually transmitted infections.
   c. stress, abuse, inadequate housing, inadequate education.
   d. miscarriage, hypothyroidism, poor weight gain.

8. Women over the age of 35 who desire a pregnancy are at increased risk for:

   a. congenital anomalies.
   b. infertility.
   c. diabetes.
   d. hypertension.
   e. all of the above.

9. Sexually transmitted infections place the pregnant woman at risk for:

   a. infertility.
   b. premature rupture of membranes.
   c. preterm labour.
   d. preterm delivery.
   e. all of the above.
   f. b, c, and d only.

10. Abdominal pain in the first trimester may be indicative of:

   a. preterm labour.
   b. ectopic pregnancy.
   c. appendicitis.
   d. urinary tract infection.
   e. all of the above.
   f. b, c, and d.

11. A woman at approximately 20 weeks' gestation who is complaining of lower right or left quadrant pain, or both, may be experiencing:

   a. appendicitis.
   b. constipation.
   c. urinary tract infection.
   d. stretching of the round ligament.
   e. none of the above.

12. You are palpating the maternal abdomen at approximately 35 weeks. Your left hand is on the maternal right, and your right hand is on the maternal left. What manoeuvre is this?

   a. Leopold's first manoeuvre
   b. Leopold's second manoeuvre
   c. Schmidt's third manoeuvre
   d. Schmidt's second manoeuvre

13. Fetal heart tones are best auscultated over the fetal:

   a. back.
   b. abdomen.
   c. shoulder.

14. Chadwick's sign is:

   a. softening of the cervix.
   b. rotation of the cervix to the left.
   c. fundus of the uterus tips forward.
   d. a bluish colour of the cervix and vaginal walls during early pregnancy.

15. An obstetric ultrasound is done to determine:

    a. thickness of the uterine wall.

    b. fetal position.

    c. placental location.

    d. amniotic fluid volume.

    e. none of the above.

    f. b, c, and d.

16. Write a narrative account of some abnormal findings in pregnancy. List possible causes and consequences to the mother and fetus.

SKILLS LABORATORY/CLINICAL SETTING

You are now ready for the clinical component of the pregnant female examination. Because of the need to maintain personal privacy, it is unlikely you will practise this examination on a peer. Some clinical settings may arrange for pregnant women to participate, or your practice setting may have available a pregnant teaching mannequin that you may use to practise your skills. If you have a pregnant woman available, discuss with her, in the presence of your instructor, the methods of examination that will be used. Maintain her comfort and adequate positioning to prevent maternal dizziness, nausea, and hypotension, and to maintain adequate uterine blood flow.

CLINICAL OBJECTIVES

1. Demonstrate the knowledge of the physical changes related to pregnancy in the first, second, and third trimesters.

2. Demonstrate the knowledge and importance of obtaining a pertinent health history during the first prenatal visit.

3. Demonstrate cultural sensitivity during the examination.

4. Inspect and palpate the maternal abdomen for uterine size and fetal position.

5. Demonstrate obtaining fetal heart tones.

6. Record the history and physical examination findings accurately, reach an assessment of the health state, estimated gestational age, and fetal position (when appropriate), and develop a plan of care.

INSTRUCTIONS

Prepare the examination setting and gather your equipment. Collect the health history before the woman disrobes for the examination. Calculate the EDD. Wash your hands. Practise the steps of the examination on a woman in the clinical setting, giving appropriate instructions and explanations as you proceed. Record your findings using the regional write-up sheet that follows. The first section is intended as a worksheet; the last page is intended for your narrative summary recording using the SOAP format. See Chapter 26 for the female genital examination.

_____
Patient Name   Date

PRENATAL HISTORY QUESTIONNAIRE

Having a healthy baby is a special event. Once a baby is born, families take certain precautions to ensure the baby's health and safety. The unborn child deserves similar care.

QUESTIONNAIRE

The following questions will help in the care of your pregnancy. Please answer these questions as well as you can. All answers will remain private. If you need help answering the questions, please ask your healthcare provider. The first question relates to your family history. The next seven questions will be about you, your baby's father, and both your families. When thinking about your families, please include your child (or unborn baby), mother, father, sisters, brothers, grandparents, aunts, uncles, nieces, nephews, or cousins.

Yes   No   1.   Will you be 35 years or older when the baby is due? Age when due: _____ .

Yes   No   2.   Are you and the baby's father related to each other (e.g., cousins)?

Yes   No   3.   Have you had three or more pregnancies that ended in miscarriage?

Yes   No   4.   Have you or the baby's father had a stillborn baby or a baby who died around the time of delivery?

Yes   No   5.   Do either you or the baby's father have a birth defect or genetic condition such as a baby born with an open spine (spina bifida), a heart defect, or Down syndrome?

Yes   No   6.   Does anyone in your family or anyone in the baby's father's family have a birth defect or condition that has been diagnosed as genetic or inherited, such as open spine (spina bifida), a heart defect, or Down syndrome?

Yes   No   7.   Where your ancestors came from may sometimes give us important information about the health of your baby. Are you or the baby's father from any of the following ethnocultural groups: Jewish, African, Asian, Mediterranean (Greek, Italian)?

Yes   No   8.   Have you or the baby's father ever been screened to see if you are carriers of the gene for any of the following: Tay-Sachs, sickle cell, thalassemia?

Sometimes, the unborn baby can be exposed to outside factors that can cause birth defects. The next eight questions will give us important information about possible exposure to the baby.

Yes   No   9.   Have you had any X-rays during this pregnancy?

Yes   No   10.   Have you had any alcohol during this pregnancy?

11.   Prior to your pregnancy, how often did you drink alcoholic beverages?
☐ Every day   ☐ Less than once a month
☐ At least once a week, not daily   ☐ I do not drink alcoholic beverages.
☐ At least once a month, not weekly

12.   Prior to your pregnancy, about how many alcoholic beverages did you usually have per occasion? (1 = one can of beer, one wine cooler, one glass of wine, or one shot of liquor.)
☐ 3 or more
☐ 1 to 2
☐ I do not drink alcoholic beverages.

Yes   No   13.   Have you taken any over-the-counter, prescription, or "street" drugs during this pregnancy? If yes, list drugs.

_____

_____

Yes   No   14.   Have you ever sought or received treatment for alcohol or drug problems? If yes, how long ago?_____

Yes   No   15.   Do you think you are at increased risk of having a baby with a birth defect or genetic disorder?

Yes   No   16.   At any time during the first two months of your pregnancy, have you had a rash or a fever of 39.4°C or greater?

A test for HIV is strongly recommended for all pregnant women, regardless of your responses to the next questions. The test is voluntary. There are two reasons to be tested: [1] New medications are available to reduce the chance of an infected mother passing HIV to her baby; and [2] most women do not know if they are infected with HIV until late in the disease. Sometimes other infections can put you and your baby at risk. The following questions will help your healthcare provider determine other areas for counselling and evaluation.

Yes   No   Unsure   17.   Have you or your sexual partners ever had a sexually transmitted infection (STI or VD) such as chlamydia, gonorrhea, syphilis, or herpes?

Yes   No   Unsure   18.   Have you ever had a serious pelvic infection or pelvic inflammatory disease (PID)?

Yes   No   Unsure   19.   Do you think any of your male sexual partners have ever had sex with other men?

Yes   No   Unsure   20.   Have you or your sexual partners ever used IV street drugs?

Yes   No   Unsure   21.   Have you had sex with two or more partners in the last 12 months?

Yes   No   Unsure   22.   Do you think any of your sexual partners may have HIV or AIDS?

Yes   No   Unsure   23.   Have you or your sexual partners ever had a blood transfusion?

How safe you feel in your daily living gives us important information about risks to you and your baby. Please answer these questions as well as you can. All answers will remain private.

                    24.   Do you feel safe....
Yes   No   -   in your personal relationship?
Yes   No   -   within your home?
Yes   No   -   in your own neighbourhood?
Yes   No   -   other (specify)_____

Yes   No   25.   Have you ever had your feelings repeatedly hurt, been repeatedly put down, or experienced other kinds of hurting?

Yes   No   26.   Are you being or have you ever been hit, slapped, kicked, pushed, or otherwise physically hurt? If yes, by whom?
☐ Husband   ☐ Family member
☐ Ex-husband   ☐ Stranger
☐ Partner   ☐ Other (specify)_____

Yes   No   27.   Are you experiencing or have you ever experienced uncomfortable touching or forced sexual contact? If yes, by whom?
☐ Husband   ☐ Family member
☐ Ex-husband   ☐ Stranger
☐ Partner   ☐ Other (specify)_____

RM/603 REV 6/97

PRENATAL RECORD

DATE	AGE	ETHNICITY	RELIGION	OCCUPATION	YRS. ED.	MARITAL STATUS	FATHER OF BABY	FATHER'S WORK PHONE

PHONE-HOME	PHONE-WORK	ADDRESS	REFERRAL-SOURCE	MOTHER'S PRIMARY CARE PROVIDER

GYNECOLOGICAL HISTORY / MEDICAL HISTORY - CONTINUED

GYNECOLOGICAL HISTORY		MEDICAL HISTORY - CONTINUED	
MENARCHE ___ YRS	INTERVAL ☐ REGULAR ☐ IRREGULAR	CARDIOVASCULAR	
DURATION ___ DAYS		RESPIRATORY/TB	
✔ IF NEGATIVE-DESCRIBE POSITIVE HISTORY		GI	
PAP HISTORY		GU	
INFERTILITY		METABOLIC	
GYN DISORDER		NEURO	
GYN SURGERY		PSYCH-EMOTIONAL	
DES EXPOSURE		HEPATITIS	
PRIOR CONTRACEPTION		MUSCULOSKELETAL	
BCP W/IN 90 DAYS CONCEP		SKIN DISORDERS	
BREASTS		OTHER DISEASE/DX	
OTHER GYN HX		OPERATIONS	
GONORRHEA		TRANSFUSIONS	
SYPHILIS		ALLERGIES	
CHLAMYDIA		FAMILY HISTORY - NOTE IF FATHER OF BABY	
HERPES-SELF/PARTNER		DIABETES	
OTHER STI/HIV		HYPERTENSION	
MEDICAL HISTORY		TWINS	
✔ IF NEGATIVE-DESCRIBE POSITIVE HISTORY		CONGENITAL ANOM	
HEENT		OTHER FAMILY HX	

PREVIOUS PREGNANCIES

NO.	DATE	LENGTH (WKS)	LABOUR (HRS)	TYPE DELIVERY	ANAES.	SEX	WEIGHT	WHERE DELIVERED	COMPLICATIONS-AP, IP, PP, NEONATAL	OUTCOME/ NAME

PRESENT PREGNANCY HISTORY / PHYSICAL EXAMINATION

PRESENT PREGNANCY HISTORY		PHYSICAL EXAMINATION	DATE
LMP ☐ NORM ☐ ABNORM	LNMP	✔ IF NEGATIVE-DESCRIBE POSITIVE FINDINGS	
EDC	+ PG TEST TYPE DATE	HEIGHT	
PLANNED PREGNANCY/OK?	FATHER SUPPORTIVE?	WEIGHT	
		B.P.	
✔ IF NEGATIVE-DESCRIBE POSITIVE HISTORY		HEENT	
NAUSEA/VOMITING		NECK	
BLEEDING		LUNGS	
URINARY SX		BREASTS	
VAGINAL DISCHARGE		HEART	
INFECTION		ABDOMEN	
FEVER/RASH		NEURO	
TOBACCO/SMOKING		EXTREMITIES/SKIN	
ETOH		PELVIC EXAMINATION	DATE
PHYSICAL/SEXUAL ABUSE		EXT. GENITALIA	
		VAGINA/CERVIX	
PATIENT NO.		UTERUS-SIZE	
		PELVIS	
		ADNEXA	
PATIENT NAME		BONY PELVIS/ADEQUATE?	
		HEMORRHOIDS	
D.O.B.		PROVIDER SIGNATURE	

FIRST TRIMESTER DATE	WEEKS	EDC/RANGE	DATE	PROBLEMS AND RISK FACTORS
LMP				
LNMP				
OVU/CONCEP				
FIRST EXAM				
+ HCG URINE				
+ HCG SERUM				
FHT DOPPLER				
FHT FETOSCOPE				
FM				
ULTRASOUND				
ULTRASOUND				
ULTRASOUND				

ANTICIPATORY GUIDANCE

FIRST TRIMESTER	SECOND TRIMESTER	THIRD TRIMESTER

CLINIC PROCEDURES/OUTLINE PRENATAL CARE
HIV COUNSELLING/TESTING
NUTRITION
VITAMINS/MINERALS
DENTAL/VISION CARE
WEIGHT GAIN
SEAT BELTS
EXERCISE
PRENATAL DIAGNOSIS
HAZARDS: SMOKING, ETOH, DRUGS, OVERHEATING, CATS,
  RAW MEAT, UNPASTEURIZED MILK
DISCOMFORTS/RELIEF MEASURES
WARNING SIGNS: BLEEDING, CRAMPS, ABDOMINAL
  PAINS, DYSURIA, ETC.
BROCHURES
	FETAL DEVELOPMENT/QUICKENING
	FAMILY/FATHER/SIBLINGS
	HOSPITAL PRE-ADMISSION/TOUR?
	FEEDING PLANS (BREAST/BOTTLE)
	EXERCISES/BODY MECHANICS
	WARNING SIGNS: SROM, BLEEDING, PRE-TERM LABOUR
	BABY'S CARE PROVIDER _____
	        NEWBORN CARE/ROOMING-IN
	        CIRCUMCISION
	BROCHURES
	PRENATAL CLASSES
	SUPPORT PERSON _____
	BIRTH PLANS/OPTIONS
	SEXUALITY
		DISCOMFORTS/RELIEF MEASURES
		WARNING SIGNS
		FETAL ACTIVITY MONITORING
		LABOUR SIGNS: WHEN AND HOW TO CALL
		TRAVEL RESTRICTIONS
		LABOUR & DELIVERY ROUTINE
		ELECTRONIC FETAL MONITORING
		ANAESTHESIA/ANALGESIA
		EPISIOTOMY/PERINEAL INTEGRITY
		LABOUR & DELIVERY COMPLICATIONS/OPERATIVE DELIVERY
		BREAST CARE
		CAR SEAT
		DISCUSS POST-TERM MANAGEMENT
		EARLY DISCHARGE/HELP AT HOME

DATE	MEDICATIONS	POSTPARTUM CONTRACEPTIVE PLANS	
	RHOGAM	☐ ORAL CONTRACEPTION	☐ LONG-ACTING CONTRACEPTION
		☐ STERILIZATION - DATE TUBAL FORM SIGNED _____	
		☐ BARRIER	☐ OTHER
DRUG ALLERGIES/REACTIONS	☐ NKA		
PATIENT NAME			
			(Continued on page 296)

(Continued on page 296)

LABORATORY DATA

TYPE RH		RUBELLA	SEROLOGY	HBsAg	HIV	URINE			DIABETIC SCREEN ___ @ ___ WKS		SICKLE PREP	PPD/TINE

ANTIBODY SCREEN	HCT		HSV SEROLOGY I _____ II _____		CERVICAL CULTURES		DATE	GTT @ ___ WKS	OTHER
___ @ ___ WKS	___ @ ___ WKS		MSAFP / MOM		CHLAMYDIA			FBS	
					GC			1 HR _____	
___ @ ___ WKS	___ @ ___ WKS		PAP	DATE	HSV			2 HR _____	COPY SENT _____
					STREP			3 HR _____	COPY SENT _____

EDC	REVISED EDC	REVISED EDC	AGE	GRAVIDA	PARA		ABORTIONS			DEATHS		LIVING CHILDREN
					TERM	PRETERM	SPONT	ELEC	ECTOPIC	FETAL	NEONATAL	

WEIGHT AND FUNDAL HEIGHT GRAPH

DATE																						
WEEKS GESTATION	6	8	10	12	14	16	18	20	22	24	26	28	30	32	33	34	35	36	37	38	39	40	41	42	43

PRENATAL VISITS

WEIGHT NON PG ___																								
BLOOD PRESSURE																								
BLOOD PRESSURE RE-CHECK																								
URINE PROTEIN/ GLUCOSE																								
FHR D-DOPPLER F-FETOSCOPE																								
PRESENTATION																								
ESTIMATE UTERINE SIZE																								
FETAL ACTIVITY																								

WEEKS GESTATION	6	8	10	12	14	16	18	20	22	24	26	28	30	32	33	34	35	36	37	38	39	40	41	42	43
FUTURE PARAMETERS TO CHECK						M S A F P OR TRIPLE SCREEN					HCT DIABETIC SCREEN RhNEG - ANTIBODY SCREEN ? RHOGAM												FETAL SURVEILLANCE		
SEE NOTE (✔)																								
RETURN WEEKS																								
INITIALS																								

PATIENT NO.   HOSPITAL

PATIENT NAME

D.O.B.

RISK FACTOR GUIDELINES	PROGRESS NOTES *(Continued from page 294)*

PATIENT PROFILE
AGE > 34 OR PREGNANCY WITHIN 2 YEARS OF MENARCHE
OCCUPATION AND AVOCATION
DRUG ABUSE OR ADDICTION
   ALCOHOL
   SMOKING
   COCAINE
   MARIJUANA
   NARCOTICS
   SEDATIVES/HYPNOTICS
   SALICYLATES AND OTHER PGSI'S
   OTHER
LOW SOCIO-ECONOMIC STATUS
   WELFARE
   EDUCATION < 9TH GRADE
   CROWDED LIVING CONDITIONS
   OTHER
BODY HABITUS
   SMALL STATURE (<152 CM TALL)
   OBESE (> 50# OVER IDEAL WEIGHT FOR HEIGHT)
   UNDERWEIGHT (> 23 KG UNDER IDEAL WEIGHT FOR HEIGHT)
   MATERNAL BIRTHWEIGHT (LOW BIRTHWEIGHT OR LARGE FOR DATES)
PARTNER
   MEDICAL OR SURGICAL DISORDERS
   DRUG, SMOKING OR ALCOHOL ABUSE
   OCCUPATION, AVOCATION, HOBBIES
   STD'S (HERPES, URETHRITIS)
   HIV RISK FACTORS

GYNECOLOGICAL HISTORY
UTERINE AND CERVICAL ABNORMALITIES
   PAST UTERINE SURGERY (NON-CESAREAN)
   UTERINE ANOMALIES (CONGENITAL ANOMALIES, DES STIGMATA, MYOMATA)
   CERVICAL LACERATIONS OR CONIZATIONS
MENSTRUAL HISTORY AND GESTATIONAL DATING
   IRREGULAR MENSES OR OLIGOAMENORRHEA
   ORAL CONTRACEPTIVE USE PRIOR TO CONCEPTION

MEDICAL HISTORY
ANEMIA (HGB <12 G/DL)
HEART DISEASE (SYMPTOMATIC OR ASYMPTOMATIC)
THROMBOEMBOLISM (DURING PREVIOUS PREGNANCY OR PRIOR TO
   CURRENT PREGNANCY)
ANTICOAGULANT USE
CHRONIC HYPERTENSION (BP > 140/90 AT FIRST PRENATAL VISIT)
ASTHMA OR OTHER CHRONIC LUNG DISEASE
SEIZURE DISORDER (WITH OR WITHOUT ANTICONVULSANT USE)
DIABETES MELLITUS (GESTATIONAL OR PREGESTATIONAL)
HEPATITIS
HIV RISK FACTORS
CHRONIC RENAL DISEASE (BUN > 20, CREATININE > 1.2 AT FIRST PRENATAL
   VISIT)
PYELONEPHRITIS

OBSTETRICAL FACTORS
PARITY
   PRIMIGRAVIDA
   GRAND MULTIPARA (> 4)
PAST PREGNANCIES
   HABITUAL ABORTION (≥ 3)
   PREMATURE BIRTH (< 37 WEEKS)
   PREMATURE RUPTURE OF MEMBRANES
   LOW BIRTH WEIGHT INFANT (BIRTHWEIGHT < 10TH PERCENTILE FOR DATES)
   LARGE FOR DATES INFANT (BIRTHWEIGHT > 90TH PERCENTILE FOR DATES)
   FETAL OR NEONATAL DEATH
   CONGENITAL ANOMALIES
   SURVIVING NEUROLOGICALLY IMPAIRED INFANT
   CERVICAL INCOMPETENCY
   MIDFORCEP OR DIFFICULT DELIVERY (E.G. SHOULDER DYSTOCIA)
   ABNORMAL LABOR (ARREST OR PROTRACTION DISORDER OF FIRST OR
     SECOND STAGE)
   ANTEPARTUM HEMORRHAGE (PLACENTAL ABRUPTION, PLACENTA PREVIA)
   BLEEDING PRIOR TO 20 WEEKS
   RH ISOIMMUNIZATION
   PREGNANCY INDUCED HYPERTENSION
   CESAREAN DELIVERY (LOW TRANSVERSE, LOW VERTICAL, CLASSICAL,
     UNKNOWN)
   INTERVAL FROM LAST DELIVERY < 12 MONTHS
   ANESTHESIA INTOLERANCE OR REACTIONS

PRESENT PREGNANCY
   EMOTIONAL STRESS
   POOR COMPLIANCE
   LATE REGISTRATION FOR CARE
   UNCERTAIN DATES
   FAILURE TO GAIN WEIGHT (< 0.25 KG PER WEEK AFTER 12 WEEKS)
   EXCESSIVE WEIGHT GAIN (> 0.9 KG PER WEEK AFTER 12 WEEKS)
   BLEEDING PRIOR TO 20 WEEKS
   LACK OF PREGNANCY NAUSEA AND VOMITING (MORNING SICKNESS)
   PLACENTAL ABRUPTION
   PLACENTA PREVIA
   OTHER VAGINAL BLEEDING
   PREMATURE RUPTURE OF MEMBRANES
   POLYHYDRAMNIOS OR OLIGOHYDRAMNIOS
   THREATENED PREMATURE LABOR

PATIENT NAME

RM 612 REV 5/97

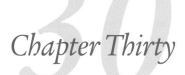

Chapter Thirty

Functional Assessment of the Older Adult

GLOSSARY

Study the following terms after completing the reading assignment. You should be able to cover the definitions on the right and define the term out loud

Activities of daily living ....tasks that are necessary for self-care, such as eating or feeding, bathing, grooming, toileting, walking, and transferring

Advanced activities of daily living ....activities that an older adult performs as a family member or as a member of society or community, including occupational and recreational activities

Caregiver assessment ....assessment of the health and well-being of an individual's caregiver

Caregiver burden ....the perceived strain by the person who cares for an older, chronically ill, or disabled person

Domains of cognition ....domains included in mental status assessments, such as attention, memory, orientation, language, visuospatial skills, and higher cognitive functions

Elder abuse..................................a term used to describe one or more of the following situations: physical abuse, sexual abuse, emotional or psychological abuse, financial or material exploitation, abandonment, neglect, or a combination of these

Environmental assessment ....assessment of an individual's home environment and community system, including hazards in the home

Functional ability......................the ability of a person to perform activities necessary to live in modern society; may include driving, using the telephone, or performing personal tasks such as bathing and toileting

Functional assessment...............a systematic assessment that includes assessment of an individual's activities of daily living, instrumental activities of daily living, and mobility

Functional status.......................a person's actual performance of activities and tasks associated with current life roles (as defined by Richmond and colleagues)

**Instrumental activities
of daily living** ....functional abilities necessary for independent community living, such as shopping, meal preparation, housekeeping, laundry, managing finances, taking medications, and using transportation

**Katz Index of Independence
in Activities of Daily Living**.......an instrument that is used to measure physical function in older adults and the chronically ill

**Lawton Instrumental
Activities of Daily Living**...........an instrument that is used to measure an individual's ability to perform instrumental activities of daily living; it may assist in assessing one's ability to live independently

**Physical performance
measures** ....tests that measure balance, gait, motor coordination, and endurance

Social domain ....the domain that focuses on an individual's relationships within family, social groups, and the community

Social networks ....informal supports that are accessed by older adults, such as family members and close friends, neighbours, church societies, neighbourhood groups, and senior centres

Spiritual assessment ....assessment of an individual's spiritual health

STUDY GUIDE

After completing the reading assignment, you should be able to answer the following questions in the spaces provided.

1. Explain the differences between functional ability and functional status.

2. Differentiate the following and provide at least three examples of each:

    a. Activities of daily living (ADLs)

    b. Instrumental activities of daily living (IADLs)

    c. Advanced activities of daily living (AADLs)

3. Describe at least two instruments that may be used to assess the following:

    a. ADLs

    b. IADLs

    c. physical performance

4. What are the disadvantages of self-answered ADL and IADL instruments?

5. What are the advantages and disadvantages of instruments that measure physical performance?

6. Discuss at least two disorders that may alter an older adult's cognition.

7. What are some indications of possible caregiver burnout?

8. List at least three reasons that elder abuse is not reported or recognized.

9. Describe at least four findings that may indicate a need for further assessment for elder abuse.

10. List at least five risk factors for elder abuse.

11. Explain the best way to document findings in cases of suspected elder abuse.

12. Define an environmental assessment and list at least four common environmental hazards that may be found in an individual's home.

13. Discuss the best approach when performing a spiritual assessment.

14. Describe special considerations that may affect the assessment of an older adult's functional status.

15. State the priority when assessing an older adult who is in pain.

ADDITIONAL LEARNING ACTIVITIES

1. Accompany a nurse practitioner who specializes in the care of older adults as she or he makes rounds in the hospital setting or a long-term care facility.

2. In a clinical setting that focuses on older adults, such as a geriatric or psychiatric unit, a daytime geriatric psychiatric program, or a senior citizen centre, observe a nurse, occupational therapist, or social worker perform various assessments of older adults.

REVIEW QUESTIONS

This test is for you to check your own mastery of the content. Answers are provided in Appendix A.

1. An appropriate tool to assess an individual's instrumental activities of daily living would be a tool by:

   a. Katz.
   b. Lawton.
   c. Tinetti.
   d. Norbeck.

2. Which of the following statements is true regarding an individual's functional status?

   a. Functional status refers to one's ability to care for another person.
   b. An older adult's functional status is usually static over time.
   c. An older adult's functional status may vary from independence to disability.
   d. Dementia is an example of functional status.

3. An older person is experiencing an acute change in cognition. The nurse recognizes that this disorder is:

   a. Alzheimer's dementia.
   b. attention deficit disorder.
   c. depression.
   d. delirium.

4. Assessment of the social domain includes:

   a. family relationships.
   b. the ability to cook meals.
   c. the ability to balance the chequebook and pay bills.
   d. hazards found in the home.

5. An older person has extensive bruising on her back and arms. Her caregiver, who is her son, explains that she fell on the stairs. When performing an assessment, the nurse's best action would be to:

   a. ask the patient what happened in the presence of her son.
   b. arrange time to interview the elder and the son separately.
   c. notify authorities of elder abuse.
   d. document the assessment on the admission history form.

6. The nurse will use which technique when assessing an older individual who has cognitive impairment?

   a. asking open-ended questions
   b. completing the entire assessment in one session
   c. asking the family members for information instead of the older individual
   d. asking simple questions that have yes or no answers.

7. An older person needs to be assessed before going home as to whether he or she is able to go outside alone, safely. The nurse will suggest which test for this assessment?

   a. Up and Go Test
   b. Performance of Activities of Daily Living test
   c. Older Americans Resources and Services Multidimensional Functional Assessment Questionnaire (OARS)
   d. Lawton IADL instrument

8. The nurse is assessing an older adult who has a history of dementia and had surgery for a fractured hip. The nurse should keep in mind that older adults with cognitive impairment:

   a. experience less pain.
   b. can provide a self-report of pain.
   c. cannot be relied on to self-report pain.
   d. will not express pain sensations.

9. An appropriate use for the Caregiver Strain Index would be which situation?

   a. a daughter who is taking her elderly father home to live with her
   b. an older patient who lives alone
   c. a wife who has cared for her husband for the past four years at home
   d. a son whose parents live in an assisted living facility

Match column B with column A.

Column A—Examples or Indicators

10. _____ Verbal assaults, insults, or threats

11. _____ Failure to provide life necessities such as food and water

12. _____ Bruised skin and broken bones

13. _____ An elder's report of unwanted touching

14. _____ An elder's report of being left alone for long periods without adequate support

15. _____ Misusing or stealing money or possessions

Column B—Type of Elder Abuse

a. Physical abuse

b. Abandonment

c. Financial or material exploitation

d. Neglect

e. Emotional or psychological abuse

f. Sexual abuse

SKILLS LABORATORY/CLINICAL SETTING

You are now ready for the clinical component of functional assessment of the older adult. The purpose of the clinical component is to practise portions of a functional assessment either in a clinical setting with older adults (such as a geriatric inpatient unit or an assisted living facility) or in the home of an older adult (such as a neighbour or family member). In addition, the following should be achieved:

CLINICAL OBJECTIVES

1. Using the Katz Activities of Daily Living instrument, assess the ADLs of an older individual.

2. Assessing the safety of the environment of an older person by using the Keeping Your Home Safe Checklist.

INSTRUCTIONS

Katz ADL:
Review the questions on the assessment form. In a clinical setting, such as a long-term care facility or a hospital setting, use the Katz ADL form to assess at least three older individuals. Compare the results of the three assessments. Did you identify any areas of dependence? Did you actually observe the areas, or did the older adult self-report?

Home Safety Checklist:

Review the questions on the checklist, then practise the assessment in your own home. Did you identify any areas of concern? After practising at your home, perform this assessment in the home of an older adult, such as a neighbour or a family member. Review the results and provide suggestions for improving safety as indicated by the assessment.

BOX 30-6	The Public Health Agency of Canada's "Keeping Your Home Safe" Checklist

Outside:
- Do all your entrances have an outdoor light?
- Do your outdoor stairs, pathways, or decks have railings and provide good traction (i.e., textured surfaces)?
- Are the front steps and walkways around your house in good repair and free of clutter, snow, and leaves?
- Do the doorways to your balcony or deck have a low sill or threshold?
- Can you reach your mailbox safely and easily?
- Is the number of your house clearly visible from the street and well lit at night?

Inside:
- Are all rooms and hallways in your home well lit?
- Are all throw rugs and scatter mats secured in place to keep them from slipping?
- Have you removed scatter mats from the top of the stairs and high-traffic areas?
- Are your high-traffic areas clear of obstacles?
- Do you always take steps to ensure that your pets are not underfoot?
- If you use floor wax, do you use the nonskid kind?
- Do you have a first aid kit and know where it is?
- Do you have a list of emergency numbers near all phones?

Excerpts from Public Health Agency of Canada. (2005). *The safe living guide—A guide to home safety for seniors* (3rd ed.). Ottawa, ON: Minister of Public Works and Government Services Canada. Retrieved April 18, 2008, from http://www.hc-sc.gc.ca/seniors-aines/pubs/safelive/index.htm

	Katz Activities of Daily Living	
Activities Points (1 or 0)	**Independence** (1 Point) NO supervision, direction, or personal assistance	**Dependence** (0 Points) WITH supervision, direction, personal assistance, or total care
Bathing Points _____	(1 Point) Bathes self completely or needs help in bathing only a single part of the body such as the back, genital area, or disabled extremity	(0 Points) Needs help with bathing more than one part of the body or getting in or out of the tub or shower. Requires total bathing.
Dressing Points _____	(1 Point) Gets clothes from closet and drawers and puts on clothes and outer garments complete with fasteners. May have help tying shoes.	(0 Points) Needs help with dressing self or needs to be completely dressed
Toileting Points _____	(1 Point) Gets to toilet, gets on and off, arranges clothes, cleans genital area without help	(0 Points) Needs help transferring to the toilet, cleaning self, or to use bedpan or commode
Transferring Points _____	(1 Point) Moves in and out of bed or chair unassisted. Mechanical transferring aids are acceptable.	(0 Points) Needs help in moving from bed to chair or requires a complete transfer
Continence Points _____	(1 Point) Exercises complete self-control over urination and defecation	(0 Points) Is partially or totally incontinent of bowel or bladder
Feeding Points _____	(1 Point) Gets food from plate into mouth without help. Preparation of food may be done by another person	(0 Points) Needs partial or total help with feeding or requires parenteral feeding
Total points = _____	6 = High (patient independent)	0 = Low (patient very dependent)

Modified from Gerontological Society of America. Katz S, Down TD, Cash HR, & Grotz RC. (1970). Progress in the development of the index of ADL, *Gerontologist,* 10, 20–30.

Caregiver Strain Questionnaire

I am going to read a list of things that other people have found to be difficult in helping out after somebody comes home from the hospital. ***Would you tell me whether any of these apply to you?*** (Give examples)

	Yes = 1	No = 0
Sleep is disturbed (e.g., because . . . is in and out of bed or wanders around at night)		
It is inconvenient (e.g., because helping takes so much time or it's a long drive over to help)		
It is a physical strain (e.g., because of lifting in and out of a chair; effort or concentration is required)		
It is confining (e.g., helping restricts free time or cannot go visiting)		
There have been family adjustments (e.g., because helping has disrupted routine; there has been no privacy)		
There have been changes in personal plans (e.g., had to turn down a job; could not go on vacation)		
There have been emotional adjustments (e.g., because of severe arguments)		
Some behaviour is upsetting (e.g., because of incontinence; . . . has trouble remembering things; or . . . accuses people of taking things)		
It is upsetting to find . . . has changed so much from his/her former self (e.g., he/she is a different person than he/she used to be)		
There have been work adjustments (e.g., because of having to take time off)		
It is a financial strain		
Feeling completely overwhelmed (e.g., because of worry about . . .; concerns about how you will manage)		
Total Score (count yes responses)		

From Sullivan, M.T. (2002). Caregiver strain index (CSI), Try this: Best practice in nursing care to older adults: Issue #14. Retrieved from http://www.hartfordign.org/publications/trythis/issue14.pdf.

APPENDIX A

Answers to Review Questions

Chapter 1: Critical Thinking in Health Assessment

1. a	3. c	5. c
2. d	4. b	6. d

Chapter 2: Developmental Tasks and Health Promotion Across the Lifespan

1. c	5. c	9. a
2. b	6. d	10. c
3. a	7. d	11. b
4. d	8. c	

Chapter 3: Cultural and Social Considerations in Health Assessment

1. c	4. b	6. a
2. b	5. e	
3. c		

Chapter 4: The Interview

1. a	6. b	10. d
2. a	7. a	11. b
3. b	8. d	12. c
4. c	9. b	13. a
5. d		

Chapter 5: The Complete Health History

1. d	5. c	8. d
2. a	6. c	9. b
3. c	7. a	10. d
4. b		

Chapter 6: Mental Status Assessment

1. d	10. c	19. Patient is dressed and groomed appropriately for season and setting. Posture is erect, with no involuntary body movements. Oriented to time, person, and place. Recent and remote memory intact. Affect and verbal responses appropriate. Perceptions and thought processes logical and coherent.
2. a	11. i	
3. d	12. d	
4. c	13. b	
5. b	14. g	
6. c	15. f	
7. b	16. a	
8. c	17. e	
9. a	18. h	

Chapter 7: Interpersonal Violence Assessment

1. d	4. b	7. d
2. a	5. a	8. d
3. b	6. e	9. b

Chapter 8: Assessment Techniques and the Clinical Setting

1. d	4. a	7. c
2. c	5. c	8. c
3. b	6. d	

Chapter 9: General Survey, Measurement, and Vital Signs

1. d	5. c	9. d
2. c	6. a	10. a
3. b	7. b	11. d
4. a	8. b	12. c

Chapter 10: Pain Assessment: The Fifth Vital Sign

1. c	5. d	9. c
2. b	6. b	10. d
3. c	7. b	11. b
4. d	8. d	

Chapter 11: Nutritional Assessment

1. c	6. b	11. c
2. d	7. b	12. d
3. c	8. a	13. b
4. c	9. b	14. d
5. b	10. c	15. c

Chapter 12: Skin, Hair, and Nails

1. b	12. c	23. a
2. d	13. c	24. b
3. a	14. c	25. d
4. d	15. a	26. b
5. b	16. c	27. a
6. d	17. b	28. g
7. c	18. c	29. c
8. c	19. a	30. f
9. a	20. a	31. d
10. c	21. b	32. e
11. d	22. c	

Chapter 13: Head, Face, and Neck, Including Regional Lymphatics

1. d	9. a	16. h
2. c	10. a	17. g
3. b	11. a	18. i
4. a	12. c	19. j
5. d	13. c	20. b
6. d	14. e	21. d
7. c	15. f	22. a
8. d		

Chapter 14: Eyes

1. b	9. a	16. Instruct the patient to hold the head steady and follow the examiner's finger. The examiner holds the finger 30 centimetres from the individual and moves it clockwise to the positions of 2, 3, 4, 8, 9, and 10 o'clock and back to the centre each time. A normal response is parallel tracking of the object with both eyes.
2. c	10. c	
3. a	11. b	
4. b	12. c	
5. d	13. b	
6. c	14. a	
7. a	15. b	
8. c		

Chapter 15: Ears

1. c	7. c	12. a
2. a	8. d	13. b
3. d	9. b	14. b
4. b	10. d	15. a
5. a	11. b	16. d
6. c		

Chapter 16: Nose, Mouth, and Throat

1. c	5. b	9. c
2. d	6. a	10. a
3. a	7. b	11. d
4. a	8. d	12. a

Chapter 17: Breasts and Regional Lymphatics

1. d	6. c	11. c
2. b	7. c	12. b
3. a	8. c	13. d
4. c	9. b	14. a
5. b	10. d	15. b

Chapter 18: Thorax and Lungs

1. a	9. c	17. d
2. b	10. d	18. b
3. b	11. b	19. e
4. a	12. c	20. a
5. c	13. a	21. d
6. b	14. e	22. f
7. b	15. a	23. c
8. d	16. c	24. b

Chapter 19: Heart and Neck Vessels

1. c	17. f	22. The major risk factors for heart disease and stroke are hypertension, smoking, high cholesterol levels, obesity, and diabetes. Physical inactivity, family history of heart disease, and age are other risk factors.
2. b	18. a	
3. c	19. b	
4. b	20. d	
5. d	21. Liver to right atrium via inferior vena cava, through tricuspid valve to right ventricle, through the pulmonic valve to the pulmonary artery, picks up oxygen in the lungs, returns to left atrium, to left ventricle via mitral valve, through aortic valve to aorta, and out to the body.	
6. d		
7. b		
8. b		
9. a		
10. a		
11. a		
12. b		
13. c		
14. c		
15. e		
16. c		

Chapter 20: Peripheral Vascular System and Lymphatic System

1. a	6. d	11. a
2. c	7. a	12. c
3. c	8. d	13. a
4. b	9. b	14. c
5. c	10. d	

Chapter 21: The Abdomen

1. c	6. a	11. d
2. c	7. d	12. a
3. a	8. d	13. c
4. d	9. d	14. b
5. c	10. a	

Chapter 22: Musculoskeletal System

1. d
2. b
3. d
4. c
5. d
6. a
7. a
8. c
9. b

10. The musculoskeletal system provides support to the body, enabling it to stand erect and to move. The system protects inner organs, produces red blood cells, and provides for the storage of minerals.
11. b
12. e
13. g

14. i
15. d
16. a
17. j
18. m
19. k
20. n
21. l
22. h
23. f
24. c

Chapter 23: Neurological System

1. a
2. d
3. c
4. c
5. b
6. c
7. b
8. a

9. b
10. d
11. b
12. c
13. f
14. b
15. g
16. k

17. h
18. c
19. l
20. d
21. i
22. e
23. j
24. a

Chapter 24: Male Genitourinary System

1. c
2. c
3. d
4. c
5. c
6. d
7. b

8. a
9. d
10. a
11. a
12. b
13. e
14. Voids clear, amber urine five or six times a day. No nocturia, dysuria, or hesitancy. No pain or discharge from penis. Sexually active

with multiple partners. Uses prophylaxis that is satisfactory for both partners. No history of sexually transmitted disease. No lesions, inflammation, or discharge from penis noted on examination. Testes descended without masses. No inguinal hernia.

Chapter 25: Anus, Rectum, and Prostate

1. a
2. b
3. c
4. a
5. d
6. c
7. b
8. c

9. a
10. No recent change in bowel habits. One soft, dark brown BM daily. No pain or bleeding. No medications. Diet includes four servings of fruits and vegetables daily. No hemorrhoids or rectal

lesions noted. Sphincter tone good. No masses or tenderness on palpation. No masses, tenderness, or enlargement of prostate. Stool is Hematest negative.

Chapter 26: Female Genitourinary System

1. d
2. a
3. d
4. c
5. c
6. d
7. d
8. b

9. c
10. b
11. b
12. a
13. a
14. Menarche at age 14, cycle 28 to 32 days, of four to five days' duration. Flow

moderate with no dysmenor-rhea. Gravida 0/Para 0/Ab 0. Has annual gynecological examination. No urinary problems, no vaginal dis-charge. Uses barrier method of birth control. Method satis-factory to self and partner.

Chapter 29: Pregnancy

1. c
2. a
3. c
4. a
5. c
6. c
7. b
8. e
9. f
10. f
11. d
12. b
13. c

14. d
15. f
16. Possible answers include:
   a. Fundal height small for dates. Possible causes: inaccurate dates, prema-ture labour, intrauterine growth restriction, fetal position
   b. Fundal height large for dates. Possible causes: inaccurate dates, hydatidi-form mole, multiple

   fetuses, polyhydramnios, fibroids, fetal macrosomia
   c. Vaginal bleeding. Possible causes: blighted ovum, friable cervix, ectopic preg-nancy, perigestational hem-orrhage, cervical lesions, threatened miscarriage, placenta previa, abruptio placentae, uterine rupture

Chapter 30: Functional Assessment of the Older Adult

1. b
2. c
3. d
4. a
5. b
6. d
7. a
8. b

9. c
10. e
11. d
12. a
13. f
14. b
15. c

APPENDIX B

Summary of Infant Growth and Development

AGE (MOS)	PHYSICAL COMPETENCY	INTELLECTUAL COMPETENCY	EMOTIONAL-SOCIAL COMPETENCY
1 to 2	Holds head in alignment when prone; Moro reflex to loud sound; follows objects; smiles.	Reflex activity; vowel sounds produced.	Gratification through sucking and basic needs being promptly met; smiles at people.
2 to 4	Turns back to side; raises head and chest 45–90 degrees off bed and supports weight on arms; reaches for objects; follows object through midline; drools; begins to localize sounds; prefers configuration of face.	Reproduces behaviour initially achieved by random activity; imitates behaviour previously done. Visually studies objects; locates sounds; makes cooing sounds; does not look for objects removed from presence.	Social responsiveness; awareness of those who are not primary caregiver; smiles in response to familiar face.
4 to 6	Birth weight doubled; teeth eruption may begin; sits with stable head and back control; rolls from abdomen to back; picks up object with palmar grasp.	Some intentional actions; some sense of object permanence, looks on same path for vanished object; recognizes partially hidden objects; more systematic in imitative behaviour; babbles.	Prefers primary caregiver; sucking needs decrease; laughs in pleasure.
6 to 8	Turns back to stomach; sits alone; crawls; transfers objects hand to hand; turns to sound behind.	Continued development as in four to six months.	Differentiated response to nonprimary caregivers; evidence of "stranger" or "separation" anxiety.
8 to 10	Creeps; pulls to stand; pincer grasp.	Actions more goal-directed; able to solve simple problems by using previously mastered responses. Actively searches for an object that disappears.	Attachment process complete.
10 to 12	Birth weight tripled; cruises; stands by self; may use spoon.	Begins to imitate behaviour done before by others but not by self. Understands words being said; may say one to four words. Intentionality is present.	Begins to explore and separate briefly from parent.

Modified from Betz C, Hunsberger M, Wright S: *Family-Centered Nursing Care of Children,* 2nd ed. Philadelphia, Saunders, 1994, pp 148–149. Used with permission.

AGE (MOS)	NUTRITION	PLAY	SAFETY
1 to 2	Breastfed or fortified formula.	Variety of positions. Caregiver should hold and talk to infant. Large, brightly coloured objects.	Car carrier; proper use of infant seat.
2 to 4	As for one to two months.	Talk to and hold. Musical toys; rattle, mobile. Variety of objects of different colour, size, and texture; mirror, crib toys, variety of settings.	Do not leave unattended on couch, bed, etc. Remove any small objects that infant could choke on.
4 to 6	Introduction of solids; initial store of iron depletion.	Talk and hold. Provide open space to move and objects to grasp.	Keep environment free of safety hazards; check toys for sharp edges and small pieces that might break.
6 to 8	As for four to six months.	Provide place to explore. Stack toys, blocks; nursery rhymes.	

Continued

Summary of Infant Growth and Development – cont'd

AGE (MOS)	NUTRITION	PLAY	SAFETY
8 to 10	As for four to six months.	Games: hide and seek, peek-a-boo, pat-a-cake, looking at pictures in a book.	Check infant's expanding environment for hazards. Keep: electrical outlets plugged, cords out of reach, stairs blocked, coffee and end tables cleared of hazards. Do not leave alone in bathtub. Keep poisons out of reach and locked up.
10 to 12	More solids than liquids; increasing use of cup; begin to wean.	Increase space; read to infant. Name and point to body parts. Water; sand play; ball.	Continue use of safety seat in car. As for eight to ten months.

APPENDIX C

Summary of Toddler Growth, Development, and Health Maintenance

AGE (MOS)	PHYSICAL COMPETENCY	INTELLECTUAL COMPETENCY	EMOTIONAL-SOCIAL COMPETENCY

General: 1 to 3 yrs	Gains 5 kg (11 lb)
	Grows 20.3 cm (8 in)
	12 teeth erupt
	Nutritional requirements:
	  Energy 100 Kcal/kg/day
	  Fluid 115–125 mL/kg/day
	  Protein 1.8 gm/kg/day
	  See Chapter 6 for vitamins and minerals.
		Learns by exploring and experimenting.
		Learns by imitating.
		Progresses from a vocabulary of three to four words at 12 months to about 900 words at 36 months.
			Central crisis: to gain a sense of experimenting autonomy versus doubt and shame.
			Demonstrates independent behaviours. Exhibits attachment behaviour strongly and regularly until third birthday. Fears persist of strange people, objects, and places and of aloneness and being abandoned. Egocentric in play (parallel play). Imitation of parents in household tasks and activities of daily living.

15 mos	Legs appear bowed. Walks alone, climbs, slides downstairs backward. Stacks two blocks. Scribbles spontaneously. Grasps spoon but rotates it, holds cup with both hands. Takes off socks and shoes.	Trial and error method of learning. Experiments to see what will happen. Says at least three words. Uses expressive jargon.	Shows independence by trying to feed self and helps in undressing.
18 mos	Runs but still falls. Walks upstairs with help. Slides downstairs backwards. Stacks three to four blocks. Clumsily throws a ball. Unzips a large zipper. Takes off simple garments.	Begins to maintain a mental image of an absent object. Concept of object permanence fully develops. Has vocabulary of 10 or more words. Holophrastic speech (one word used to communicate whole ideas).	Fears the water. Temper tantrums may begin. Negativism and dawdling predominate. Bedtime rituals begin. Awareness of gender identity begins. Helps with undressing.

From Betz C, Hunsberger M, Wright S: *Family-Centered Nursing Care of Children*, 2nd ed. Philadelphia, Saunders, 1994, pp 190–191. Used with permission.

Continued

Summary of Toddler Growth, Development, and Health Maintenance—cont'd

AGE (MOS)	PHYSICAL COMPETENCY	INTELLECTUAL COMPETENCY	EMOTIONAL-SOCIAL COMPETENCY
24 mos	Runs quickly and with fewer falls. Pulls toys and walks sideways. Walks downstairs hanging on a rail (does not alternate feet). Stacks six blocks. Turns pages of a book. Imitates vertical and circular strokes. Uses spoon with little spilling. Can feed self. Puts on simple garments. Can turn door knobs.	Enters into preconceptual phase of preoperational period: Symbolic thinking and symbolic play. Egocentric thinking, imagination, and pretending are common. Has vocabulary of about 300 words. Uses two-word sentences (telegraphic speech). Engages in monologue.	Fears the dark and animals. Temper tantrums may continue. Negativism and dawdling continue. Bedtime rituals continue. Sleep resisted overtly. Usually shows readiness to begin bowel and bladder control. Explores genitalia. Brushes teeth with help. Helps with dressing and undressing.
36 mos	Has set of deciduous teeth at about 30 months. Walks downstairs alternating feet. Rides tricycle. Walks with balance and runs well. Stacks eight to ten blocks. Can pour from a pitcher. Feeds self completely. Dresses self almost completely (does not know front from back). Cannot tie shoes.	Preconceptual phase of preoperational period as for 24 months. Uses around 900 words. Constructs complete sentences and uses all parts of speech.	Temper tantrums subside. Negativism and dawdling subside. Bedtime rituals subside. Self-care in feeding, elimination, and dressing enhances self-esteem.

	NUTRITION	PLAY	SAFETY
General: 1 to 3 yrs	Milk 16–24 oz. Appetite decreases. Wants to feed self. Has food jags. Never force food; give nutritious snacks. Give iron and vitamin supplementation only if poor intake.	Books at all stages. Needs physical and quiet activities, does not need expensive toys.	Never leave alone in tub. Keep poisons, including detergents and cleaning products, out of reach. Use car seat.
15 mos	Vulnerable to iron deficiency anemia. Give table foods except for tough meat and hard vegetables. Wants to feed self.	Stuffed animals, dolls, music toys. Peek-a-boo, hide and seek. Water and sand play. Stacking toys. Roll ball on floor. Push toys on floor. Read to toddler.	Keep small items off floor (pins, buttons, clips). Child may choke on hard food. Cords and tablecloths are a danger. Keep electrical outlets plugged and poisons locked away. Risk of kitchen accidents with toddler underfoot.
18 mos	Negativism may interfere with eating. Encourage self-feeding. Is easily distracted while eating. May play with food. High activity level interferes with eating.	Rocking horse. Nesting toys. Shape-sorting cube. Pencil or crayon. Pull toys. Four-wheeled toy ride. Throw ball. Running and chasing games. Roughhousing. Puzzles. Blocks. Hammer and peg board.	Falls: from riding toy, in bathtub, from running too fast. Climbs up to get dangerous objects. Keep dangerous things out of waste-basket.
24 mos	Requests certain foods; therefore snacks should be controlled. Imitates eating habits of others. May still play with food and especially with utensils and dish (pouring, stacking).	Clay and Play-Doh. Finger paint. Brush paint. Music player with story book and songs to sing along. Toys to take apart. Toy tea sets. Puppets. Puzzles.	May fall from outdoor large play equipment. Can reach farther than expected (knives, razors, and matches must be kept out of reach).
36 mos	Sits in booster seat rather than high chair. Verbal about likes and dislikes.	Likes playing with other children, building toys, drawing and painting, doing puzzles. Imitation household objects for doll play. Nurse and doctor kits. Carpenter kits.	Protect from turning on hot water, falling from tricycle, striking matches.

APPENDIX D

Growth, Development, and Health Promotion for Preschoolers

AGE (YRS)	PHYSICAL COMPETENCY	INTELLECTUAL COMPETENCY	EMOTIONAL-SOCIAL COMPETENCY

General: 3 to 5	Gains 4.5 kg (10 lb)
	Grows 15 cm (6 in)
	20 teeth present
	Nutritional requirements:
	  Energy: 1250 to 1600 cal/day
	  (or 90 to 100 Kcal/kg/day)
	  Fluid: 100 to 125 mL/kg/day
	  Protein: 30 g/day (or 3 g/kg/day)
	  Iron: 10 mg/day
		Becomes increasingly aware of self and others. Vocabulary increases from 900 to 2100 words.
		Piaget's preoperational/intuitive period.
			Freud's phallic stage
			  Oedipus complex—boy.
			  Electra complex—girl.
			Erikson's stage of Initiative vs. Guilt.

3	Runs, stops suddenly. Walks backward. Climbs steps. Jumps. Pedals tricycle. Undresses self. Unbuttons front buttons. Feeds self well.	Knows own sex. Sense of humour. Desires to please. Language—900 words. Follows simple direction. Uses plurals. Names figure in picture. Uses adjectives and adverbs.	Shifts between reality and imagination. Bedtime rituals. Negativism decreases. Animism and realism: anything that moves is alive.
4	Runs well, skips clumsily. Hops on one foot. Heel-toe walks. Up and down steps without holding rail. Jumps well. Dresses and undresses. Buttons well, needs help with zippers, bows. Brushes teeth. Bathes self. Draws with some form and meaning.	More aware of others. Uses alibis to excuse behaviour. Bossy. Language—1500 words. Talks in sentences. Knows nursery rhymes. Counts to five. Highly imaginative. Name calling.	Focuses on present. Egocentrism; unable to see the view point of others, unable to understand another's inability to see own viewpoint. Does not comprehend anticipatory explanation. Sexual curiosity. Oedipus complex. Electra complex.
5	Runs skillfully. Jumps three to four steps. Jumps rope, hops, skips. Begins dance. Roller skates. Dresses without assistance. Ties shoelaces. Hits nail on head with hammer. Draws person—six parts. Prints first name.	Aware of cultural differences. Knows name and address. More independent. More sensible, less imaginative. Copies triangle, draws rectangle. Knows four or more colours. Language—2100 words, meaningful sentences. Understands kinship. Counts to ten.	Continues in egocentrism. Fantasy and daydreams. Resolution of Oedipus/Electra complex, girls identify with mother, boys with father. Body image and body boundary especially important in illness. Shows tension in nail-biting, nose-picking, whining, snuffling.

From Betz C, Hunsberger M, Wright S: *Family-Centered Nursing Care of Children*, 2nd ed. Philadelphia, Saunders, 1994, pp 235–236. Used with permission.

Continued

Growth, Development, and Health Promotion for Preschoolers – cont'd

		NUTRITION	PLAY	SAFETY
General: 3 to 5		Carbohydrate intake approximately 40 to 50 percent of calories. Good food sources of essential vitamins and minerals. Regular tooth brushing. Parents are seen as examples; if parent will not eat it, neither will the child.	Reading books is important at all ages. Balance highly physical activities with quiet times. Quiet rest period takes the place of nap time. Provide sturdy play materials.	Never leave alone in bath or swimming pool. Keep poisons in locked cupboard; learn what household things are poisonous. Use car seats and seatbelts. Never leave child alone in car. Remove doors from abandoned refrigerators.
3		1250 Kcal/day. Due to increased sex identity and imitation, copies parents at table and will eat what they eat. Different colours and shapes of foods can increase interest.	Participates in simple games. Cooperates, takes turns. Plays with group. Uses scissors, paper. Likes crayons, colouring books. Enjoys being read to and "reading." Plays "dress-up" and "house." Likes fire engines.	Teach safety habits early. Let water out of bathtub; don't stand in tub. Caution against climbing in unsafe areas, onto or under cars, unsafe buildings, drainage pipes. Insist on seatbelts worn at all times in cars.
4		Good nutrition. 1400 Kcal/day. Nutritious between-meal snacks essential. Emphasis on quality not quantity of food eaten. Mealtime should be enjoyable, not for criticism. As dexterity improves, neatness increases.	Longer attention span with group activities. "Dress-up" with more dramatic play. Draws, pounds, paints. Likes making paper chains, sewing cards. Scrapbooks. Likes being read to, listening to music, and rhythmic play. "Helps" adults.	Teach to stay out of streets, alleys. Continually teach safety; child understands. Teach how to handle scissors. Teach what are poisons and why to avoid. Never allow child to stand in moving car.
5		Good nutrition. 1600 Kcal/day. Encourage regular tooth brushing. Encourage quiet time before meals. Can learn to cut own meat. Frequent illnesses from increased exposure increase nutritional needs.	Plays with trucks, cars, soldiers, dolls. Likes simple games with letters or numbers. Much gross motor activity: water, mud, snow, leaves, rocks. Matching picture games.	Teach chid how to cross streets safely. Teach child not to speak to strangers or get into cars of strangers. Insist on seatbelts. Teach child to swim.

APPENDIX E

Competency Development of the School-Age Child

AGE (YRS)	PHYSICAL COMPETENCY	INTELLECTUAL COMPETENCY	EMOTIONAL-SOCIAL COMPETENCY
General: 6 to 12	Gains an average of 2.5 to 3.2 kg/year (5 1/2 to 7 lbs/year). Overall height gains of 5.5 cm (2 in) per year; growth occurs in spurts and is mainly in trunk and extremities. Loses deciduous teeth; most of permanent teeth erupt. Progressively more coordinated in both gross and fine motor skills. Caloric needs increase with growth spurts.	Masters concrete operations. Moves from egocentrism; learns he or she is not always right. Learns grammar and expression of emotions and thoughts. Vocabulary increases to 3000 words or more; handles complex sentences.	Central crisis: industry vs. inferiority; wants to do and make things. Progressive sex education needed. Wants to be like friends; competition important. Fears body mutilation, alterations in body image; earlier phobias may recur, nightmares; fears death. Nervous habits common.
6 to 7	Gross motor skill exceeds fine motor coordination. Balance and rhythm are good—runs, skips, jumps, climbs, gallops. Throws and catches ball. Dresses self with little or no help.	Vocabulary of 2500 words. Learning to read and print; beginning concrete concepts of numbers, general classification of items. Knows concepts of right and left; morning, afternoon, and evening; coinage. Intuitive thought process. Verbally aggressive, bossy, opinionated, argumentative. Likes simple games with basic rules.	Boisterous, outgoing, and a know-it-all, whiney; parents should sidestep power struggles, offer choices. Becomes quiet and reflective during seventh year; very sensitive. Can use telephone. Likes to make things: starts many, finishes few. Give some responsibility for household duties.
8 to 10	Myopia may appear. Secondary sex characteristics begin in girls. Hand-eye coordination and fine motor skills well established. Movements are graceful, coordinated. Cares for own physical needs completely. Constantly on move; plays and works hard; enforce balance in rest and activity.	Learning correct grammar and to express feelings in words. Likes books he or she can read alone; will read comics, scan newspaper. Enjoys making detailed drawings. Mastering classification, seriation, spatial and temporal, numerical concepts. Uses language as a tool; likes riddles, jokes, chants, word games. Rules guiding force in life now. Very interested in how things work, what and how weather, seasons, etc., are made.	Strong preference for same-sex peers; antagonizes opposite-sex peers. Self-assured and pragmatic at home; questions parental values and ideas. Has a strong sense of humour. Enjoys clubs, group projects, outings, large groups, camp. Modesty about own body increases over time; sex conscious. Works diligently to perfect skills he or she does best. Happy, cooperative, relaxed, and casual in relationships. Increasingly courteous and well-mannered with adults. Gang stage at a peak; secret codes and rituals prevail. Responds better to suggestion than dictatorial approach.
11 to 12	Vital signs approximate adult norms. Growth spurt for girls; inequalities between sexes are increasingly noticeable; boys have greater physical strength. Eruption of permanent teeth complete except for third molars. Secondary sex characteristics begin in boys. Menstruation may begin.	Able to think about social problems and prejudices; sees others' points of view. Enjoys reading mysteries, love stories. Begins playing with abstract ideas. Interested in whys of health measures and understands human reproduction. Very moralistic; religious commitment often made during this time.	Intense team loyalty; boys begin teasing girls and girls flirt with boys for attention; best friend period. Wants unreasonable independence. Rebellious about routine; wide mood swings; needs some time daily for privacy. Very critical of own work. Hero worship prevails. "Facts of life" chats with friends prevail; masturbation increases. Appears under constant tension.

From Betz C, Hunsberger M, Wright S; *Family-Centered Nursing Care of Children,* 2nd ed. Philadelphia, Saunders, 1994, pp 281–282. Used with permission.

Continued

Competency Development of the School-Age Child – cont'd

	NUTRITION	PLAY	SAFETY
General: 6 to 12	Fluctuations in appetite due to uneven growth pattern and tendency to get involved in activities. Tendency to neglect breakfast owing to rush of getting to school. Though school lunch is provided in most schools, child does not always eat it.	Plays in groups, mostly of same sex; "gang" activities predominate. Books for all ages. Bicycles important. Sports equipment. Cards, board and table games. Most of play is active games requiring little or no equipment.	Enforce continued use of safety belts during car travel. Bicycle safety must be taught and enforced. Teach safety related to hobbies, handicrafts, mechanical equipment.
6 to 7	Preschool food dislikes persist. Tendency for deficiencies in iron, vitamin A, and riboflavin. 100 mL/kg of water per day. 3 g/kg protein daily.	Still enjoys dolls, cars, and trucks. Plays well alone but enjoys small groups of both sexes; begins to prefer same sex peer during seventh year. Ready to learn how to ride a bicycle. Prefers imaginary, dramatic play with real costumes. Begins collecting for quantity, not quality. Enjoys active games such as hide-and-seek, tag, jumprope, roller skating, kickball. Ready for lessons in dancing, gymnastics, music. Restrict TV time to one to two hours per day.	Teach and reinforce traffic safety. Still needs adult supervision of play. Teach to avoid strangers, never take anything from strangers. Teach illness prevention and reinforce continued practice of other health habits. Restrict bicycle use to home ground; no traffic areas; teach bicycle safety. Teach the harmful use of drugs, alcohol, smoking. Set a good example.
8 to 10	Needs about 2100 calories per day; nutritious snacks. Tends to be too busy to bother to eat. Tendency for deficiencies in calcium, iron, and thiamine. Problem of obesity may begin now. Good table manners. Able to help with food preparation.	Likes hiking, sports. Enjoys cooking, woodworking, crafts. Enjoys cards and table games. Likes radio and music. Begins qualitative collecting now. Continue restriction on TV time.	Stress safety with firearms. Keep them out of reach and allow use only with adult supervision. Know who the child's friends are; parents should still have some control over friend selection. Teach water safety; swimming should be supervised by an adult.
11 to 12	Male needs 2500 calories per day; female needs 2250 (70 Kcal/kg/day). 75 mL/kg of water per day. 2 g/kg protein daily.	Enjoys projects and working with hands. Likes to do errands and jobs to earn money. Very involved in sports, dancing, talking on phone. Enjoys all aspects of acting and drama.	Continue monitoring friends; stress bicycle safety on streets and in traffic.

APPENDIX F

Characteristics of Adolescents

EARLY ADOLESCENCE (12 TO 14 YR)	MIDDLE ADOLESCENCE (15 TO 16 YR)	LATE ADOLESCENCE (17 TO 21 YR)
Becomes comfortable with own body; egocentric.	"Tries out" adultlike behaviour.	Aware of own strengths and limitations; establishes own value system.
Difficulty solving problems; thinks in present; cannot use past experience to control behaviour; sense of invulnerability— society's rules do not apply to him or her.	Begins to solve problems, analyze, and abstract. Established peer group alliance with associated risk-taking behaviour.	Able to verbalize conceptually: deals with abstract moral concepts; makes decisions regarding future.
Struggle between dependent and independent behaviour; begins forming peer alliance.	Peak turmoil in child–family relations; able to debate issues and use some logic but not continuously.	Peer group diminishes in importance; may develop first intimate relationship.
Parent–child conflict begins; teen argues, but without logic.		Turbulence subsides. May move away from home. More adultlike friendship with parents.

From Foster R, Hunsberger M, Anderson JJ: *Family-Centered Nursing Care of Children*. Philadelphia, Saunders, 1989, p. 359. Used with permission.

APPENDIX G

Functional Health Patterns Guide

The following table is a general guide for programs employing a functional health patterns approach to assessment.

Functional Health Patterns	Potential Correlating Chapters in the Text
Health Perception—Health Management	• Chapter 2, Developmental Tasks and Health Promotion Across the Lifespan • Chapter 4, The Interview • Chapter 5, The Complete Health History • Chapter 30, Functional Assessment of the Older Adult
Nutritional—Metabolic	• Chapter 11, Nutritional Assessment • Chapter 9, General Survey, Measurement, and Vital Signs • Chapter 12, Skin, Hair, and Nails • Chapter 16, Nose, Mouth, and Throat • Chapter 21, The Abdomen
Elimination	• Chapter 21, The Abdomen • Chapter 24, Male Genitourinary System • Chapter 25, Anus, Rectum, and Prostate • Chapter 26, Female Genitourinary System
Activity—Exercise	• Chapter 18, Thorax and Lungs • Chapter 19, Heart and Neck Vessels • Chapter 20, Peripheral Vascular System and Lymphatic System • Chapter 22, Musculoskeletal System
Sleep—Rest	• Chapter 5, The Complete Health History
Cognitive—Perception	• Chapter 6, Mental Status Assessment • Chapter 10, Pain Assessment: The Fifth Vital Sign • Chapter 13, Head, Face, and Neck, Including Regional Lymphatics • Chapter 14, Eyes • Chapter 15, Ears • Chapter 16, Nose, Mouth, and Throat • Chapter 23, Neurological System • Chapter 30, Functional Assessment of the Older Adult
Self-Perception—Self-Concept	• Chapter 2, Developmental Tasks and Health Promotion Across the Lifespan • Chapter 6, Mental Status Assessment • Chapter 30, Functional Assessment of the Older Adult
Role—Relationship	• Chapter 2, Developmental Tasks and Health Promotion Across the Lifespan • Chapter 3, Cultural and Social Considerations in Health Assessment • Chapter 7, Interpersonal Violence Assessment • Chapter 30, Functional Assessment of the Older Adult
Sexuality—Reproductive	• Chapter 17, Breasts and Regional Lymphatics • Chapter 24, Male Genitourinary System • Chapter 26, Female Genitourinary System • Chapter 29, Pregnancy
Coping—Stress Tolerance	• Chapter 2, Developmental Tasks and Health Promotion Across the Lifespan • Chapter 30, Functional Assessment of the Older Adult
Values—Beliefs	• Chapter 2, Developmental Tasks and Health Promotion Across the Lifespan • Chapter 3, Cultural and Social Considerations in Health Assessment